OXFORD MEDICAL PUBLICATIONS

Health Measurement Scales

A Practical Guide to their Development and Use

Health Measurement Scales

A Practical Guide to their Development and Use

David L. Streiner

and

Geoffrey R. Norman

Department of Clinical Epidemiology and Biostatistics,
McMaster University

OXFORD · NEW YORK · TOKYO
OXFORD UNIVERSITY PRESS
1989

Oxford University Press, Walton Street, Oxford OX2 6DP
Oxford New York Toronto
Delhi Bombay Calcutta Madras Karachi
Petaling Jaya Singapore Hong Kong Tokyo
Nairobi Dar es Salaam Cape Town
Melbourne Auckland
and associated companies in
Berlin Ibadan

Oxford is a trade mark of Oxford University Press

Published in the United States
by Oxford University Press, New York

British Library Cataloguing in Publication Data
Streiner David L.
Health measurement scales
1. Man. Health. Assessment
I. Title II. Norman Geoffrey R.
613
ISBN 0–19–261773–7

Library of Congress Cataloging in Publication Data
Streiner, David L.
Health measurement scales.
(Oxford medical publications)
Bibliography: p.
Includes indexes.
1. Health surveys.   2. Health status indicators—
Measurement.   3. Public health—Evaluation   4. Medical
care—Evaluation.   I. Norman, Geoffrey R.   II. Title.
III. Series.
RA408.5.S77   1989   362.1   89–16103
ISBN 0–19–261773–7

Set by
Promenade Graphics, Cheltenham
and printed in Great
Britain by Biddles Ltd,
Guildford and King's Lynn

Contents

1

Introduction

The act of measurement is an essential component of scientific research, whether in the natural, social, or health sciences.

Until recently, however, discussion regarding issues of measurement was noticeably absent in the deliberations of clinical researchers. Certainly, measurement played as essential a role in research in the health sciences as in other scientific disciplines. However, measurement in the laboratory disciplines presented no inherent difficulty. Like other natural sciences, measurement was a fundamental part of the discipline, and was approached through the development of appropriate instrumentation. Subjective judgement played a minor role in the measurement process; any issue of reproducibility or validity was therefore amenable to a technological solution. It should be mentioned, however, that expensive equipment does not, of itself, eliminate measurement error.

Conversely, clinical researchers were acutely aware of the fallibility of human judgement as evidenced by the errors involved in such processes as radiological diagnosis (Garland 1959; Yerushalmy 1955). Fortunately the research problems approached by many clinical researchers—cardiologists, epidemiologists, and the like—frequently did not depend on subjective assessment. Trials of therapeutic regimens focused on the prolongation of life and the prevention or management of such life-threatening conditions as heart disease, stroke, or cancer. In these circumstances, measurement is reasonably straightforward. 'Objective' criteria, based on laboratory or tissue diagnosis where possible, can be used to decide whether a patient has the disease, and warrants inclusion in the study. The investigator then waits an appropriate period of time and counts those who did or did not survive—and the criteria for death are reasonably well established, even though the exact cause of death may be a little more difficult.

In the past decade or so, the situation in clinical research has become more complex. The effects of new drugs or surgical procedures on *quantity* of life is likely to be marginal indeed. Conversely, there is increased awareness of the impact of health and health care on the *quality* of human life. Therapeutic efforts in many disciplines of medicine—psychiatry, respirology, rheumatology, oncology—other health professions—nursing, physiotherapy, occupational therapy—are directed equally if not primarily to the improvement of quality, not quantity of life. If the efforts of these disciplines are to be placed on a sound scientific basis, methods must be devised to measure what was previously thought to be unmeasurable, and assess in a reproducible and valid fashion those subjective states which cannot be converted into the position of a needle on a dial.

The challenge is not as formidable as it may seem. Psychologists and educators have been grappling with the issue for many years, dating back to the European attempts at the turn of the century to assess individual differences in intelligence (Galton 1979; Stern 1979). Since that time, and particularly since the 1930s, much has been accomplished, so that a sound methodology for the development and application of tools to assess subjective states now exists. Unfortunately, much of this literature is virtually unknown to most clinical researchers. Health Science libraries do not routinely catalog *Psychometrica* or *The British Journal of Statistical Psychology*. Nor should they—the language would be incomprehensible to most readers, and the problems of seemingly little relevance.

Similarly, the textbooks in the subject are directed at educational or psychological audiences. The former is concerned with measures of achievement applicable to classroom situations, and the latter is focused primarily on personality or aptitude measures, again with no apparent direct relevance. In general, textbooks in these disciplines are directed to the development of achievement, intelligence or personality tests.

By contrast, researchers in health sciences are frequently faced with the desire to measure something which has not been approached previously—arthritic pain, return to function of post-MI patients, speech difficulties of aphasic stroke patients, or clinical competence of junior medical students. The difficulties and questions raised in developing such instruments range from the straightforward (e.g. 'How many boxes do I put on the response?') to the complex (e.g. 'How do I establish whether the thing is measuring what I hope it is?'). Nevertheless, to a large degree, the answers are known, although frequently difficult to access.

The intent of this book is to introduce researchers in health sciences to these concepts of measurement. It is not an introductory textbook, in that we do not confine ourselves to a discussion of introductory principles and methods; rather, we attempt to make the book as current and comprehensive as possible. The book does not delve as heavily into mathematics as many books in the field; such side trips may provide some intellectual rewards for those so inclined, but frequently at the expense of losing the majority of readers. Similarly, we emphasize applications, rather than theory, so that some theoretical subjects (like Thurstone's Law of Comparative Judgement) which are of historical interest but little practical importance, are omitted. Nevertheless, we spend considerable time in explanation of the concepts underlying current approaches to measurement. One other departure from current books is that our focus is on those attributes of interest to researchers in health sciences—subjective states, attitudes, response to illness, etc. rather than the topics such as personality or achievement familiar to readers in education and psychology. As a result, our examples are drawn from the literature in health sciences.

Finally, some understanding of certain selected topics in statistics is necessary to learn many essential concepts of measurement. In particular, the *correlation coefficient* is used in many empirical studies of measurement instruments. Discussion of reliability is based on the methods of *repeated measures analysis of variance*. Item analysis and certain approaches to test validity use the methods of *factor analysis*. It is not by any means necessary to have detailed knowledge of these methods to understand the concepts of measurement discussed in this book. Still, it would be useful to have some conceptual understanding of these techniques. If the reader requires some review of statistical topics, we have suggested a few appropriate resources in Appendix A.

The book is organized in a sort of chronological sequence; that is, we are attempting to cover topics in the order they might be confronted by someone faced with the problem of developing a new instrument. Chapter 2 provides an overview of the criteria which should be used to assess any measurement instrument; by reviewing this section, the reader should be able to peruse the literature to see if any available instrument is suitable. In the remaining chapters, we assume an unsuccessful search, and provide detailed information regarding the steps involved in developing a new scale. Finally, the appendices provides additional resources for locating further information about issues in measurement, including an annotated bibliography of references for existing scales (Appendix B).

References

Galton, F. (1979). Cited in M. J. Allen and W. M. Yen, *Introduction to Measurement Theory*. Brooks Cole, Monterey.

Garland, L. H. (1959). Studies on the accuracy of diagnostic procedures. *American Journal of Roentgenology*, **82**, 25–38.

Stern, W. (1979). Cited in M. J. Allen and W. M. Yen, *Introduction to Measurement Theory*. Brooks Cole, Monterey.

Yerushalmy, J. (1955). Reliability of chest radiography in diagnosis of pulmonary lesions. *American Journal of Surgery*, **89**, 231–40.

2

Basic concepts

One feature of the health sciences literature devoted to measuring subjective states is the daunting array of available scales. Whether one wishes to measure depression, pain, or patient satisfaction, it seems that every article published in the field has used a different approach to the measurement problem. This proliferation impedes research, since there are significant problems in generalizing from one set of findings to another.

Paradoxically, if you proceed a little further in the search for existing instruments to assess a particular concept, you may conclude that none of the existing scales is quite right, so it is appropriate to embark on the development of one more scale to add to the confusion in the literature. Most researchers tend to magnify the deficiencies of existing measures and underestimate the effort required to develop an adequate new measure. Of course, scales do not exist for all applications; if this were so, there would be little justification for writing this book. Nevertheless, perhaps the most common error committed by clinical researchers is to dismiss existing scales too lightly, and embark on the development of a new instrument with an unjustifiably optimistic and naive expectation that they can do better. As will become evident, the development of scales to assess subjective attributes is not easy and requires considerable investment of both mental and fiscal resources. Therefore, a useful first step is to be aware of any existing scales which might suit the purpose. The next step is to understand and apply criteria for judging the usefulness of a particular scale. In subsequent chapters, these will be described in much greater detail for use in developing a scale; however, the next few pages will serve as an introduction to the topic and a guideline for a critical literature review.

The discussion which follows is necessarily brief. A much more comprehensive set of standards, which is widely used for the assessment of standardized tests used in psychology and education, is the manual called *Standards for educational and psychological tests*, published by the American Psychological Association (1985).

Searching the literature

An initial search of the literature to locate scales for measurement of particular variables might begin with the standard bibliographic sources, particularly Medline. However, depending on the application, one might wish to consider bibliographic reference systems in other disciplines, particularly *Psychological Abstracts* for psychological scales and ERIC for instruments designed for educational purposes.

In addition to these standard sources, there are a number of compendia of measuring scales. These are described in Appendix B. We might particularly highlight the volume entitled *Measuring health: A guide to rating scales and questionnaires* (McDowell and Newell 1987) which is a critical review of scales designed to measure a number of characteristics of interest to researchers in the health sciences, such as pain, illness behaviour, and social support.

Critical review

Having located one or more scales of potential interest, it remains to choose whether to use one of these existing scales or to proceed to development of a new instrument. In part this decision can be guided by a judgement of the appropriateness of the items on the scale, but this should always be supplemented by a critical review of the evidence in support of the instrument. The particular dimensions of this review are described below:

Face and content validity

The terms *face validity* and *content validity* are technical descriptions of the judgement that a scale looks reasonable. Face validity simply indicates whether, on the face of it, the instrument appears to be assessing the desired qualities. The criterion represents a subjective judgement based on a review of the measure itself by one or more experts, and rarely are any empirical approaches used. Content validity is a closely related concept, consisting of a judgement whether the instrument samples all the relevant or important content or domains. These two forms of validity consist of a judgement by experts whether the scale appears appropriate for the intended purpose. Guilford (1954) calls this approach to validation 'validity by assumption', meaning the instrument measures such-and-such because an expert says it does. However, an explicit statement regarding face and content validity, based on some form of review by an expert panel or alternative methods described later, should be a minimum prerequisite for acceptance of a measure.

Having said this, there are situations where face and content validity may not be desirable, and may be consciously avoided. For example, in assessing behaviour such as child abuse or excessive alcohol consumption, questions like 'Have you ever hit your child with a blunt object?' or 'Do you frequently drink to excess?' may have face validity, but are unlikely to elicit an honest response. Questions designed to assess sensitive areas are likely to be less obviously related to the underlying attitude or behaviour, and may appear to have poor face validity. It is rare for scales not to satisfy minimal standards of face and content validity, unless there has been a deliberate attempt from the outset to avoid straightforward questions.

Nevertheless, all too frequently, researchers dismiss existing measures on the basis of their own judgements of face validity—they did not like some of the questions, or the scale was too long, or the responses were not in a preferred format. As we have indicated, this judgement should comprise only one of several used in arriving at an overall judgement of usefulness, and should be balanced against the time and cost of developing a replacement.

Reliability

The concept of *reliability* is, on the surface, deceptively simple. Before one can obtain evidence that an instrument is measuring what is intended, it is first necessary to gather evidence that the scale is measuring *something* in reproducible fashion. That is, a first step in providing evidence of the value of an instrument is to demonstrate that measurements of individuals on different occasions, or by different observers, or by similar or parallel tests, produce the same or similar results.

That is the basic idea behind the concept—an index of the extent to which measurements of individuals obtained under different circumstances yield similar results. However, the concept is refined a bit further in measurement theory. If we were considering the reliability of, for example, a set of bathroom scales, it might be sufficient to indicate that the scales are accurate to ± 1 kg. From this information, we can easily judge whether the scales will be adequate to distinguish among adult males (probably yes) or to assess weight gain of premature infants (probably no), since we have prior knowledge of the average weight and variation in weight of adults and premature infants.

Such information is rarely available in the development of subjective scales. Each scale produces a different measurement from every other. Therefore, to indicate that a particular scale is accurate to ± 3.4 units provides no indication of its value in measuring individuals unless we have some idea about the likely range of scores on the scale. To circumvent this problem, reliability is usually quoted as a ratio of the variability between individuals to the total variability in the scores; in other words, the reliability is a measure of the proportion of the variability in scores which was due to true differences between individuals. Thus, the reliability is expressed as a number between 0 and 1, with 0 indicating no reliability, and 1 indicating perfect reliability.

An important issue in examining the reliability of an instrument is the manner in which the data were obtained which provided the basis for the calculation of a reliability coefficient. First of all, since the reliability involves the ratio of variability between subjects to total variability, one way to ensure that a test will look good is to conduct the study on an extremely hetergeneous sample, for example to measure knowledge of clinical medicine using samples of first year, third year, and fifth year students. Examine the sampling procedures carefully, and assure yourself that the sample used in the reliability study is approximately the same as the sample you wish to study.

Secondly, there are any number of ways in which reliability measures can be obtained, and the magnitude of the reliability coefficient will be a direct reflection of the particular approach used. Some broad definitions are described below:

1. *Internal consistency*. Measures of internal consistency are based on a single administration of the measure. If the measure has a relatively large number of items addressing the same underlying dimension; for example, 'Are you able to dress yourself?', 'Are you able to shop for groceries?', 'Can you do the sewing?' as measures of physical function, then it is reasonable to expect that scores on each item would be correlated with scores on all other items. This is the idea behind measures of internal consistency—essentially, they represent the average of the correlations among all the items in the measure. There are a number of ways to calculate these correlations, called *Cronbach's alpha*, *Kuder–Richardson*, or *split halves*, but all yield similar results. Since the method involves only a single administration of the test, such coefficients are easy to obtain. However, they do not take into account any variation from day to day or from observer to observer, and thus lead to an optimistic interpretation of the true reliability of the test.

2. *Stability*. There are a variety of ways of examining the reproduceability of a measure administered on different occasions. For example, one might ask about the degree of agreement between different observers (*inter-observer reliability*); the agreement between observations made by the same rater on two different occasions (*intra-observer reliability*); observations on the patient on two occasions separated by some interval of time (*test–retest reliability*), and so forth. As a minimum, any decision regarding the value of a measure should be based on some information regarding stability of the instrument. Internal consistency, in its many guises, is not a sufficient basis upon which to make a reasoned judgement.

3. *Standards of acceptable reliability*. One difficulty with the reliability coef-

ficient is that it is simply a number between 0 and 1, and does not lend itself to commonsense interpretations. Various authors have made different recommendations regarding the minimum accepted level of reliability. Certainly, internal consistency should exceed 0.8, and it might be reasonable to demand stability measures greater than 0.5. Depending on the use of the test, and the cost of misinterpretation, higher values might be required.

Finally, although there is a natural concern that many instruments in the literature are too long to be practical, the reason for the length should be borne in mind. If we assume that every response has some associated error of measurement, then by averaging or summing responses over a series of questions, we can reduce this error. For example, if the original test has a reliability of 0.5, doubling the test will increase the reliability to 0.67, and quadrupling it will result in a reliability of 0.8. As a result, we must recognize that there is a very good reason for long tests; brevity is not necessarily a desirable attribute of a test, and is achieved at some cost.

Empirical forms of validity

Reliability simply assesses that a test is measuring something in a reproducible fashion; it says nothing about *what* is being measured. To determine that the test is measuring what was intended requires some evidence of 'validity'. To demonstrate validity requires more than peer judgements; empirical evidence must be produced to show that the tool is measuring what is intended. How is this achieved?

Although there are many approaches to assessing validity, and myriad terms used to describe these approaches, eventually the situation reduces to two circumstances:

1. *Other scales of the same or similar attributes are available.* In the situation where measures already exist, then an obvious approach is to administer the experimental instrument and one of the existing instruments to a sample of people and see whether there is a strong correlation between the two. As an example, there are many scales to measure depression. In developing a new scale, it is straightforward to administer the new and old instruments to the same sample. This approach is described by several terms in the literature including *convergent validity*, *criterion validity*, and *concurrent validity*. The distinction among the terms will be made clear in Chapter 10.

Although this method is straightforward it has two severe limitations. First, if other measures of the same property already exist, then it is difficult to justify developing yet another unless it is cheaper or simpler. Of course, many researchers believe that the new instrument that they are developing is better than the old, which provides an interesting bit of circular logic. If the new method is better than the old, why compare it to the old method? And if the relationship between the new method and the old is less than perfect, which one is at fault?

In fact, the nature of the measurement challenges we are discussing in this book usually precludes the existence of any conventional 'gold standard'. Although there are often measures which have, through history or longevity, acquired criterion status, a close review usually suggests that they have less than ideal reliability and validity. Any measurement we are likely to make will have some associated error; as a result we should expect that correlations among measures of the same attribute should fall in the midrange of 0.4–0.8. Any lower correlation suggests that either the reliability of one or the other measure is likely unacceptably low, or that they are measuring different phenomena.

2. *No other measure exists.* This situation is the more likely, since it is usually the justification for developing a scale in the first instance. At first glance, though, we seem to be confronting an impossible situation. After all, if no measure exists, how can one possibly acquire data to show that the new measure is indeed measuring what is intended?

The solution lies in a broad set of approaches labelled *construct validity*. We begin by linking the attribute we are measuring to some other attribute by a hypothesis or construct. Usually this hypothesis will explore the difference between two or more populations who would be expected to have differing amounts of the property assessed by our instrument. We then test this hypothetical construct by applying our instrument to the appropriate samples. If the expected relationship is found, then the hypothesis and the measure are sound; conversely, if no relationship is found, the fault may lie with either the measure or the hypothesis.

Let us clarify this with an example. Suppose that the year is 1920, and a biochemical test of blood sugar has just been devised. Enough is known to hypothesize that diabetics have higher blood sugar values than normal subjects; but no other test of blood sugar exists. Here are some likely hypotheses which could be tested empirically:

- Individuals diagnosed as diabetic on clinical criteria will have higher blood sugar on the new test than comparable controls.
- Dogs whose pancreases are removed will show increasing levels of blood sugar in the days from surgery until death.
- Individuals who have sweet-tasting urine will have higher blood sugar than those who do not.
- Diabetics injected with insulin extract will show a decrease in blood sugar levels following the injection.

These hypotheses certainly do not exhaust the number of possibilities, but each can be put to an experimental test. Further, it is evident that we should not demand a perfect relationship between blood sugar and the other variable, or even that each and all relationships are significant. But the weight of the evidence should be in favour of a positive relationship.

Similar constructs can be developed for almost any instrument, and in the absence of a concurrent test, some evidence of construct validity should be available. However, the approach is non-specific, and is unlikely to result in very strong relationships. Therefore, the burden of evidence in testing construct validity arises not from a single powerful experiment, but from a series of converging experiments.

Summary

The criteria we have described are intended as a guideline for reviewing the literature, and as an introduction to the remainder of this book. We must emphasize that the research enterprise involved in development of a new method of measurement requires time and patience. Effort expended to locate an existing measure is justified, because of the savings if one can be located and the additional insights provided in the development of a new instrument if none prove satisfactory.

References

American Psychological Association (1985). *Standards for educational and psychological testing*. American Psychological Association, Washington.
Guilford, J.P. (1954). *Psychometric methods*. McGraw-Hill, New York.
McDowell, I. and Newell, C. (1987). *Measuring health*. Oxford University Press, Oxford.

3

Devising the items

The first step in writing a scale or questionnaire is, naturally, devising the items themselves. This is far from a trivial task, since no amount of statistical manipulation after the fact can compensate for poorly chosen questions; those that are badly worded, ambiguous, irrelevant, or—even worse—not present. In this chapter we explore various sources of items, and the strengths and weaknesses of each of them.

The first step is to look at what others have done in the past. Instruments rarely spring full grown from the brows of their developers. Rather, they are usually based on what other people have deemed to be relevant, important, or discriminating. Wechsler (1958), for example, quite openly discussed the patrimony of the subtests which were later incorporated into his various IQ tests. Of the 11 subtests which comprise the adult version, at least nine were derived from other widely used indices. Moreover, the specific items which make up the individual subtests are themselves based on older tests. Both the items and the subtests were modified and new ones added to meet his requirements, but in many cases the changes were relatively minor. Similarly, the *Manifest Anxiety Scale* (Taylor 1953) is based in large measure on one scale from the *Minnesota Multiphasic Personality Inventory* (MMPI; Hathaway and McKinley 1951).

However, the motivation for developing a new tool is the investigator's belief that the previous scales are inadequate for one reason or another, or do not completely cover the domain under study. At this point, new items can come from four different sources: clinical observation, theory, research, or expert opinion, although naturally the lines between these categories are not firm.

The source of items

Clinical observation is perhaps one of the most fruitful sources of items. Indeed, it can be argued that observation, whether of patients or students, precedes theory, research, or expert opinion. Scales are simply a way of gathering these clinical observations in a systematic fashion, so that all observers are ensured of looking for the same thing, or all subjects of responding to the same items. As an example, Kruis *et al.* (1984) devised a scale to try to differentiate between irritable bowel syndrome (IBS) and organic bowel disease. The first part of their questionnaire consists of a number of items asked by the clinician of the patient—presence of abdominal pain and flatulence, alteration in bowel habits, duration of symptoms, type and intensity of pain, abnormality of the stools, and so forth. The choice of these items was predicated on the clinical experience of the authors, and their impressions of how IBS patients' symptomatology and presentation differ from other patients'. Similarly, the *Menstrual Distress Questionnaire* (Moos 1984) consists of 47 symptoms, such as muscle stiffness, skin blemishes, fatigue, and feeling sad or blue, which have been reported clinically to be associated with premenstrual syndrome (PMS).

This is not to say that these groups of researchers are necessarily correct, in that the items they selected *are* different between patients with organic or functional bowel disease, or between women who do and do not have PMS. In fact, perhaps the major drawback of relying solely on clinical observation to guide the selection of items is the real possibility that the clinicians may be wrong. The original rationale for electroconvulsive shock therapy, for instance, was based on a quite erroneous 'observation' that the incidence of epilepsy is far lower in the schizophrenic population than with normals. Any scale which tried to capitalize on this association would be doomed to failure. A related problem is that the clinician, because of a limited sample of patients, or narrow perspective imposed by a particular model of the disorder, may not be aware of other factors which may prove to be better descriptors or discriminators.

Clinical observation rarely exists in isolation. Individual laboratory results or physical findings convey far more information if they are components of a more global theory of an illness or behaviour. The term *theory*, in this context, is used very broadly, encompassing not only formal, refutable models of how things relate to one another, but also to vaguely formed hunches of how or why people behave, if only within a relatively narrow domain. A postulate that patients who believe in the efficacy of therapy will be more compliant with their physician's orders, for example, may not rival the theory of relativity in its scope or predictive power, but can be a fruitful source of items in this limited area. A theory or model can thus serve a heuristic purpose, suggesting items or subscales.

At first glance, it may appear as if theory is what we rely on until data are available; once studies have been done, it would be unnecessary to resort to theory and the scale developer can use facts to generate items or guide construction of the scale. Indeed, this was the prevailing attitude among test designers until relatively recently. However, there has been an increasing appreciation of the role that theory can play in scale and questionnaire development. This is seen most clearly when we are trying to assess attitudes, beliefs, or traits. For example, if we wanted to devise a scale which could predict those post-MI patients who would comply with an exercise regimen, our task would be made easier (and perhaps more accurate) if we had some model or theory of compliance. The Health Belief Model (Becker *et al*. 1979), for instance, postulates that compliance is a function of numerous factors, including the patient's perception of the severity of the disorder and his susceptibility to it, and his belief in the effectiveness of the proposed therapy, as well as external cues to comply and barriers which may impede compliance. If this model has any validity, then it would make sense for the scale to include items from each of these areas, some of which may not have occurred to the investigator without the model.

The obverse side is that a model which is wrong can lead us astray, prompting us to devise questions which ultimately have no predictive or explanatory power. While the inadequacy of the theory may emerge later in testing the validity of the scale, much time and effort can be wasted in the interim. For example, Patient Management Problems (PMPs) were based on the supposition that physician competence is directly related to the thoroughness and comprehensiveness of the history and physical examination. The problems, therefore, covered every conceivable question that could be asked of a patient and most laboratory tests that could be ordered. The scoring system similarly reflected this theory; points were gained by being obsessively compulsive, and lost if the right diagnosis were arrived at by the 'wrong' route, one which used short cuts. While psychometrically sound, the PMPs did not correlate with any other measure of clinical competence, primarily for the reason that the model was wrong—expert physicians do not function in the way envisioned by the test developers (Feightner 1985).

Just as naked observations need the clothing of a theory, so a theory must ultimately be tested empirically. *Research findings* can be a fruitful source of items and subscales. For the purposes of scale construction, research can be of two types; a literature review of studies which have been done in the area, or new research carried out specifically for the purpose of developing the scale. In both cases, the scale or questionnaire would be comprised of items which have been shown empirically to be characteristic of a group of people, or which differentiate them from other people.

As an example of a scale based on previous research, the second part of the Kruis *et al*. (1984) scale for IBS is essentially a checklist of laboratory values and clinical history; e.g. erythrocyte sedimentation rate, leucocytosis, and weight loss. These were chosen on the basis of previous research which indicated that IBS and organic patients differed on these variables. This part of the scale, then, is a summary of empirical findings based on research done by others.

In a different domain, Ullman and Giovannoni (1964) developed a scale to measure the 'process—reactive' continuum in schizophrenia. A number of items on the questionnaire relate to marriage and parenthood, because there is considerable evidence that process schizophrenics, especially males, marry at a far lower rate than do reactive schizophrenics. Another item relates to alcohol consumption, since among schizophrenics at least, those who use alcohol tend to have shorter hospital stays than those who do not drink.

When entering into a new area, though, there may not be any research which can serve as the basis for items. Under these circumstances, it may be necessary for the scale developer to conduct some preliminary research, which can then be the source of items. For example, Brumback and Howell (1972) needed an index to evaluate the clinical effectiveness of physicians working in federal hospitals and clinics. Existing scales were inadequate or inappropriate for their purposes, and did not provide the kind of information they needed in a format which was acceptable to the raters. The checklist portion of the scale they ultimately developed was derived by gathering 2500 descriptions of critical incidents from 500 people; classifying these into functional areas; and then using various item analytic techniques (to be discussed in Chapter 6) to arrive at the final set of 37 items. While this study is unusual in its size, it illustrates two points. First, it is sometimes necessary to perform research prior to constructing the scale itself in order to determine key aspects of the domain under investigation. Second, the initial item pool is often much larger than the final set of items. Again, the size of the reduction is quite unusual in this study (only 1.5 per cent of the original items were ultimately retained), but the fact that reduction occurs is not.

The use of *expert opinion* in a given field was illustrated in a similar study by Cowles and Kubany (1959) to evaluate the performance of medical students. Experienced faculty members were interviewed to determine what they felt were the most important characteristics students should have in preparing for general practice, ultimately resulting in eight items. This appears quite similar to the first step taken by Brumback and Howell, which was labelled 'research'; indeed, the line between the two is a very fine one and the distinction somewhat arbitrary. The important point is that, in both cases, information had to be gathered prior to the construction of the scale.

There are no hard and fast rules governing the use of expert judgements: how many experts to use, how they are found and chosen, or even more important, how differences among them are reconciled. The methods by which the opinions are gathered can run the gamut from having a colleague scribble some comments on a rough draft of the questionnaire to holding a conference of recognized leaders in the field, with explicit rules governing voting. Most approaches usually fall between these two extremes; somewhere in the neighbourhood of three to ten people known to the scale developer as experts are consulted, usually individually. Since the objective is to generate as many potential items as possible for the scale, those suggested by even one person should be considered, at least in the first draft of the instrument.

The advantage of this approach is that if the experts are chosen carefully, they probably represent the most recent thinking in an area. Without much effort, the scale developer has access to the accumulated knowledge and experience of others who have worked in the field. The disadvantages may arise if the panel is skewed in some way, and does not reflect a range of opinions. Then, the final selection of items may represent one particular viewpoint, and there may be glaring gaps in the final product.

It should be borne in mind that these are not mutually exclusive methods of generating items. A scale may consist of items derived from some or all of these sources. Indeed, it would be unusual to find any questionnaire derived from only one of them.

Content validity

Once the items have been generated from these various sources, the scale developer is ideally left with far more items than will ultimately end up on the scale. In Chapter 5 we will discuss various statistical techniques to select the best items from this pool. For the moment, though, we address the converse of this, ensuring that the scale has enough items and adequately covers the domain under investigation. The technical term for this is *content validity*, although some theorists have argued that 'content relevance' and 'content coverage' would be more accurate descriptors (Messick 1980). These concepts arose from achievement testing, where students are assessed to determine if they have learned the material in a specific content area; final examinations are the prime example. With this in mind, each item on the test should relate to one of the course objectives (content relevance). Items which are not related to the content of the course introduce error in the measurement, in that they discriminate among the students on some dimension other than the one purportedly tapped by the test; a dimension that can be totally irrelevant to the test. Conversely, each part of the syllabus should be represented by one or more questions (content coverage). If not, then students may differ in some important respects, but this would not be reflected in the final score. Table 3.1 shows how these two components of content validity can be checked in a course of, for example, cardiology. Each row reflects a different item on the test, and each column a different content area. Every item is examined in turn, and a mark placed in the appropriate column(s). Although a single number

Table 3.1   *Checking content validity for a course in cardiology*

Question	Content area				
	Anatomy	Physiology	Function	. . .	Pathology
1		×			
2	×				
3			×		
4	×				
5					×
.					
.					
.					
20		×			

does not emerge at the end, as with other types of validity estimates, the visual display yields much information.

First, each item should fall into at least one content area represented by the columns. If it does not, then either that item is not relevant to the course objectives, or the list of objectives is not comprehensive. Second, each objective should be represented by at least one question; otherwise, it is not being evaluated by the test. Last, the number of questions in each area should reflect its actual importance in the syllabus. The reason for checking this is that it is quite simple to write items in some areas, and far more difficult in others. In cardiology, for example, it is much easier to write multiple-choice items to find out if the students know the normal values of obscure enzymes than to devise questions tapping their ability to deal with the rehabilitation of cardiac patients. Thus, there may be a disproportionately large number of the former items on the test and too few of the latter in relation to what the students should know. The final score, then, would not be an accurate reflection of what the instructor hoped the students would learn.

Depending on how finely one defines the course objectives, it may not be possible to assess each one, as this would make the test too long. Under these conditions, it would be necessary to *randomly sample* the domain of course objectives; that is, select them in such a way that each has an equal opportunity of being chosen. This indeed is closer to what is often done in measuring traits or behaviours, since tapping the full range of them may make the instrument unwieldy.

Although this matrix method was first developed for achievement tests, it can be applied equally well to scales measuring attitudes, behaviours, symptoms, and the like. In these cases, the columns are comprised of aspects of the trait or disorder that the investigator wants the scale to cover, rather than course objectives. Assume, for example, that the test constructor wanted to develop a new measure to determine whether living in a home insulated with urea formaldehyde foam (UFFI) leads to physical problems. The columns in this case would be those areas she felt would be affected by UFFI (and perhaps a few that should *not* be affected, if she wanted to check on a general tendency to endorse symptoms). So, based on previous research, theory, expert opinion and other sources, these may include upper respiratory symptoms, gastrointestinal complaints, skin rash, sleep disturbances, memory problems, eye irritation, and so forth. This would then serve as a check that all domains were covered by at least one question, and that there were no irrelevant items. As can be seen, content validity applies to the scale as a whole, not to the separate items individually.

Let us use a concrete example to illustrate how these various steps are put into practice. As part of a study to examine the effects of stress (McFarlane *et al.* 1980), a scale was needed to measure the amount of social support that the respondents felt they had. Although there were a number of such instruments already in existence, none met the specific needs of this project, or matched closely enough our theoretical model of social support. Thus, the first step, although not clearly articulated as such at the time, was to elucidate our *theory* of social support; what areas we wanted to tap, and which we felt were irrelevant or unnecessary for our purposes. This was augmented by *research* done in the field by other groups, indicating aspects of social support which served as buffers, protecting the person against stress. The next step was to locate *previous instruments*, and cull from them those questions or approaches which met our needs. Finally, we showed a preliminary draft of our scale to a number of highly experienced family therapists, whose *expert opinion* was formed on the basis of their years of *clinical observation*. This last step actually served two related purposes: they performed a *content validity* study, seeing if any important areas were missed by us, and also suggested additional items to fill these gaps. The final draft (McFarlane *et al.* 1981) was then subjected to a variety of reliability and validity checks, as outlined in subsequent chapters.

Translation

Although it is not directly related to the problem of devising items, translation into another language is a problem that may have to be addressed. In most large studies, especially those located in major metropolitan centres, it is quite probable that English will not be the first language of a significant proportion of respondents. This raises one of two possible alternatives, both of which have associated problems. First, such respondents can be eliminated from the study. However, this raises the possibility that the sample will then not be a representative one, and the results may have limited generalizability. The second alternative is to translate the scales and questionnaires into the languages most commonly used within the catchment area encompassed by the study.

The translation process itself is a complex one, and may introduce subtle forms of distortions into the scale. The first step consists of translating the individual items or questions into the other language. This is best done by someone who is not only fluent in both English and the target tongue, but who is also knowledgeable about the content area, and is aware of the intent of each item and of the scale as a whole. The reason is that the literal translation of phrases may convey very different meanings in the two languages; feelings, disorders, and even symptoms may not be expressed in the same manner in other cultures. For example, we generally associate the colour blue with sadness, and black with depression. In China, though, white is the colour of mourning, a shade we use to connote purity. Consequently, a literal translation of the phrase, 'I feel blue,' or 'The future looks black to me' may generate a response, but the meaning of the answer would be problematic. Similarly, Anglo-Saxons often associate mild physical discomfort with stomach problems, whereas the French would be more prone to attribute it to their liver, and Germans to their circulation.

The next step, one which is unfortunately frequently omitted, is called 'back-translation.' Another bilingual person, one who was not associated with the translation phase and again preferably knowledgeable, translates the new version back into English. If the meaning seems to have been lost or altered, then that item should go through the process again.

Once the translation is done, however, there is little assurance that the psychometric properties of the scale (i.e., its reliability and validity) have remained constant. It is therefore necessary to revalidate the instrument, as if it were a new one. For more information about the translating process, the reader should refer to Sechrest *et al.* (1972).

References

Becker, M. H., Maiman, L. A., Kirscht, J. P., Haefner, D. P., Drachman, R. H., and Taylor, D. W. (1979). Patient perception and compliance: Recent studies of the health belief model. In *Compliance in health care* (eds. R. B. Haynes and D. L. Sackett) pp. 78–109. Johns Hopkins University Press, Baltimore.

Brumback, G. B., and Howell, M. A. (1972). Rating the clinical effectiveness of employed physicians. *Journal of Applied Psychology*, **56**, 241–4.

Cowles, J. T., and Kubany, A. J. (1959). Improving the measurement of clinical performance of medical students. *Journal of Clinical Psychology*, **15**, 139–42.

Feightner, J. W. (1985). Patient management problems. In *Assessing clinical competence* (eds. V. R. Neufeld and G. R. Norman) pp. 183–200. Springer-Verlag, New York.

Hathaway, S. R., and McKinley, J. C. (1951). *Manual for the Minnesota Multiphasic Personality Inventory* (rev.). Psychological Corporation, New York.

Kruis, W., Thieme, C., Weinzierl, M., Schuessler, P., Holl, J., and Paulus, W. (1984). A diagnostic score for the irritable bowel syndrome: Its value in the exclusion of organic disease. *Gastroenterology*, **87**, 1–7.

McFarlane, A. H., Norman, G. R., Streiner, D. L., Roy, R. G., and Scott, D. J. (1980). A longitudinal study of the influence of the psychosocial environment on health status: A preliminary report. *Journal of Health and Social Behavior*, **21**, 124–33.

McFarlane, A. H., Neale, K. A., Norman, G. R., Roy, R. G., and Streiner, D. L. (1981). Methodological issues in developing a scale to measure social support. *Schizophrenia Bulletin*, **7**, 90–100.

Messick, S. (1980). Test validity and the ethics of assessment. *American Psychologist*, **35**, 1012–27.

Moos, R. H. (1984). *Menstrual distress questionnaire*. Stanford University Medical Center, Palo Alto, CA.

Sechrest, L., Fay, T. L., and Hafeez Zaidi, S. M. (1972). Problems of translation in cross-cultural research. *Journal of Cross-Cultural Psychology*, **3**, 41–56.

Taylor, J. A. (1953). A personality scale of manifest anxiety. *Journal of Abnormal and Social Psychology*, **48**, 285–90.

Ullman, L. P., and Giovannoni, J. M. (1964). The development of a self-report measure of the process-reactive continuum. *Journal of Nervous and Mental Disease*, **138**, 38–42.

Wechsler, D. (1958). *The measurement and appraisal of adult intelligence* (4th edn). Williams and Wilkins, Baltimore.

4

Scaling responses

Introduction

Having devised a set of questions using the methods outlined in the previous chapter, we must choose a method by which responses will be obtained. The choice of method is dictated, at least in part, by the nature of the question asked. For example, a question like 'Have you ever gone to church?' leads fairly directly to a response method consisting of two boxes, one labelled 'Yes' and the other 'No'. By contrast, the question 'How religious are you?' does not dictate a simple two-category response, and a question like 'Do you believe that religious instruction leads to racial prejudice?' may require the use of more subtle and sophisticated techniques to obtain valid responses.

There has been a bewildering amount of research in this area, in disciplines ranging from psychology to economics. Often the results are conflicting, and the correct conclusions are frequently counter-intuitive. In this chapter, we describe a wide variety of scaling methods, indicate their appropriate use, and make recommendations regarding a choice of methods.

Some basic concepts

In considering approaches to the development of response scales, it is helpful to first consider the kinds of possible responses which may arise. A basic division is between those responses which are categorical, such as race, religion or marital status and those which are continuous variables like haemoglobin, blood pressure, or the amount of pain recorded on a 100 mm line. A second related feature of response scales is commonly referred to as the *level of measurement*. If the response consists of named categories, such as particular symptoms, a job classification, or religious denomination, the variable is called a *nominal* variable. Ordered categories, such as staging in breast cancer, educational level (less than high school, high school diploma, some college or university, university degree, postgraduate degree) are called *ordinal* variables. By contrast, variables in which the interval between responses and constant is known are called *interval* variables, naturally. Temperature, measured in degrees Celsius or Fahrenheit, is an interval variable. Generally speaking, rating scales, where the response is on a five-point or seven-point scale, are not considered interval level measurement, since we can never be sure that the distance between 'strongly disagree' and 'disagree' is the same as between 'agree' and 'strongly agree'. However, some methods have been devised to achieve interval-level measurement with subjective scales, as will be discussed. Finally, variables where there is a meaningful zero point, so that the ratio of two responses has some meaning, are called *ratio* variables. Temperature measured in Kelvin is a ratio variable, temperature degrees in Fahrenheit or Celsius is not.

What is the significance of these distinctions? The important difference lies between nominal and ordinal data on one hand, and interval and ratio variables on the other. In the latter case, measures such as means, standard deviations, and differences among means can be interpreted and the broad class of techniques called 'parametric statistics' can therefore be used for analysis. By contrast, since it makes no sense to speak of the average religion or average sex of a sample of people, nominal and ordinal data must be considered as frequencies in individual categories, and 'non-parametric' statistics must be used for analysis. The distinction between these two types of analysis is described in any introductory statistics book, such as those listed in Appendix A.

Categorical judgements

One form of question frequently used in health sciences requires only a categorical judgement by the respondent, either as a 'yes–no' response, or as a simple check. The responses would then result in a *nominal* scale of measurement. Some examples are shown in Figure 4.1. Care must be taken to ensure that questions are written clearly and unambiguously, as discussed in Chapter 5. However, there is little difficulty in deciding on the appropriate response method.

Perhaps the most common error when using categorical questions is that they are frequently employed in circumstances where the response is not, in fact, categorical. Attitudes and behaviours often lie on a continuum. When we ask a question like 'Do you have trouble climbing stairs?', we ignore the fact that there are varying degrees of trouble. Even the best athlete might have difficulty negotiating the stairs of a skyscraper at one run without some degree of discomfort. What we wish to find out presumably, is *how much* trouble the respondent has in negotiating an ordinary flight of stairs.

Ignoring the continuous nature of many responses leads to two difficulties.

Have you ever had a chest X-ray?   yes __ no __

Which of the following symptoms are you presently experiencing?

    Headaches __
    Dizziness __
    Cough __
    Colds __
    Other   (please write in) _____

Are you able to climb the stairs?   yes __ no __

I think that people are watching me.   true __ false __

Fig. 4.1 Examples of questions requiring categorical judgments.

The first is fairly obvious: since different people may have different ideas about what constitutes a positive response to a question, there will likely be error introduced into the responses, as well as uncertainty and confusion on the part of respondents.

The second problem is perhaps more subtle. Even if all respondents have a similar conception of the category boundaries, there will still be error introduced into the measurement because of the limited choice of response levels. For example, the statement in Figure 4.2 might be responded to in one of two ways, as indicated in (a) and (b): the first method effectively reduces all positive opinions, ranging from strong to mild, to a single number, and similarly for all negative feelings. The effect is a potential loss of information and a corresponding reduction in reliability.

There are two common, but invalid, objections to the use of multiple response levels. The first is that the researcher is only interested in whether respondents agree or disagree, so it is not worth the extra effort. This argument confuses measurement with decision-making; the decision can always

---

Doctors carry a heavy responsibility

(a) agree __   disagree __

(b) strongly agree	agree	mildly agree	mildly disagree	disagree	strongly disagree
__	__	__	__	__	__

Fig. 4.2 Example of a continuous judgement.

be made after the fact by establishing a cutoff point on the response continuum, but information lost from the original responses cannot be recaptured.

A second argument is that the additional categories are only adding noise or error to the data; people cannot make finer judgements than 'agree–disagree'. Although there may be particular circumstances where this is true, in general the evidence indicates that people are capable of much finer discriminations; this will be reviewed in a later section of the chapter where we discuss the appropriate number of response steps (p. 26).

Continuous judgements

Accepting that many of the variables of interest to health care researchers are continuous rather than categorical, methods must be devised to quantify these judgements.

The approaches which we will review fall into three broad categories: *direct estimation* techniques, in which subjects are required to indicate their response by a mark on a line or check in a box; *comparative* methods, in which subjects choose among a series of alternatives which have been previously calibrated by a separate criterion group; and *econometric* methods, in which the subjects describe their preference by anchoring it to extreme states (perfect health—death).

Direct estimation methods
Direct estimation methods are designed to elicit from the subject a direct quantitative estimate of the magnitude of an attribute. The approach is usually straightforward, as in the example used above, where we asked for a response on a six-point scale ranging from 'strongly agree' to 'strongly disagree'. This is one of many variations, although all share many common features. We begin by describing the main contenders, then we will explore their advantages and disadvantages.

Visual analogue scales
The visual analogue scale (VAS) is the essence of simplicity—a line of fixed length, usually 100 mm, with anchors like 'no pain' and 'pain as bad as it could be' at the extreme ends, and no words describing intermediate positions. An example is shown in Figure 4.3. Respondents are required to place a mark, usually an 'X' or a vertical line, on the line corresponding to their perceived state. The method has been used extensively in medicine to

---

How severe has your arthritic pain been today?

pain as   no
bad as it _____ pain
could be

Fig. 4.3 The visual analogue scale (VAS).

assess a variety of constructs; pain (Huskisson 1974), mood (Aitken 1969), and functional capacity (Scott and Huskisson 1978), among many others.

The VAS has also been used for the measurement of change (Scott and Huskisson 1979). In this approach, researchers are interested in perceptions of the degree to which patients feel they have improved as a result of treatment. The strategy used is to show patients, at the end of a course of treatment, where they had marked the line prior to commencing treatment, and then asking them to indicate, by a second line, their present state. There are a number of conceptual and methodological issues in the measurement of change, by VAS or other means, which will be addressed in Chapter 11.

Proponents are enthusiastic in their writings regarding the advantages of the method over its usual rival, a scale in which intermediate positions are labelled (e.g. 'mild', 'moderate', 'severe'); however, the authors frequently then demonstrate a substantial correlation between the two methods (Downie *et al.* 1978) suggesting that the advantages are more perceived than real. One also suspects that the method provides an illusion of precision, since a number given to two decimal places (e.g. a length measured in millimetres) has an apparent accuracy of 1 per cent. Of course, although one can measure a response to this degree of precision, there is no guarantee that the response accurately represents the underlying attribute to the same degree of resolution.

The simplicity of the VAS has contributed to its popularity, although there is some evidence that patients may not find it as simple and appealing as researchers; in one study described above (Huskisson 1974), 7 per cent of patients were unable to complete a VAS, as against 3 per cent for a graphic rating scale. Some researchers in geriatrics have concluded that there may be an age effect in the perceived difficulty in using the VAS, leading to a modification of the technique. Instead of a horizontal line, they have used a vertical 'thermometer', which is apparently easier for older people to complete.

Perhaps the most serious problem with the VAS is not inherent in the scale at all. In many applications of the VAS in health sciences, the attribute of interest, such as pain, is assessed with a single scale, as in the

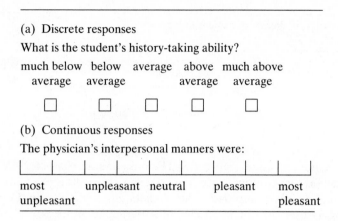

(a) Discrete responses

What is the student's history-taking ability?

much below   below   average   above   much above
   average   average   average   average

□   □   □   □   □

(b) Continuous responses

The physician's interpersonal manners were:

most   unpleasant neutral   pleasant   most
unpleasant   pleasant

Fig. 4.4 Examples of adjectival scales.

example shown earlier. However, the reliability of a scale is directly related to the number of items in the scale, so that the one-item VAS test is likely to demonstrate low reliability in comparison to longer scales. The solution, of course, is to lengthen the scale by including multiple VASs, to assess related aspects of the attribute of interest.

In conclusion, although the VAS approach has the merit of simplicity, there appears to sufficient evidence that other methods may yield more precise measurement, and possibly increased levels of satisfaction among respondents.

Adjectival scales
In contrast to the research on the VAS, most investigations in psychological rating scales have focused on scales with adjectival descriptions and discrete or continuous responses. Examples of the two approaches are shown in Figure 4.4.

It is evident that the rating scale with continuous responses bears close resemblance to the VAS, with the exception that additional descriptions are introduced at intermediate positions. Although proponents of the VAS eschew the use of descriptors, an opposite position is taken by psychometricians regarding rating scales. Guilford (1954) states 'nothing should be left undone to give the rater a clear, unequivocal conception of the continuum along which he is to evaluate objects . . . '(p. 292).

Specific scaling methods
Within this broad class of rating scales, there are several specific formats which have achieved wide popularity. One is the *Likert scale* (Likert 1952), in which the rater expresses an opinion by rating his agreement with a

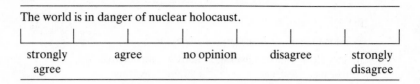

The world is in danger of nuclear holocaust.

strongly   agree   no opinion   disagree   strongly
agree   disagree

Fig. 4.5 Examples of a Likert scale.

series of statements like Figure 4.5. The only unique characteristic of the
Likert scale is that responses are framed on an agree–disagree continuum.

A second standard approach, the *semantic differential scale* (Osgood *et
al.* 1957), is used to obtain ratings of a particular object on a series of
dimensions, as shown in Figure 4.6. The basic notion is to define a number
of related dimensions of a characteristic on a series of continuous bipolar
scales.

General issues in the construction of continuous scales

Regardless of the specific approach adopted, there are a number of questions which must be addressed in designing a rating scale to maximize precision and minimize bias.

1. *How many steps should there be?* The choice of the number of steps or
boxes on a scale is not primarily an aesthetic issue. We indicated earlier in
the discussion of categorical ratings that the use of two categories to
express an underlying continuum will result in a loss of information. The
argument can be extended to the present circumstances; if the number of
levels is less than the rater's ability to discriminate, the result will be a loss
of information.

Although the ability to discriminate would appear to be highly con-
tingent on the particular situation, there is evidence that this is not the
case. A number of studies have shown that for reliability coefficients in the
range normally encountered, from 0.4 to 0.9, the reliability drops as fewer

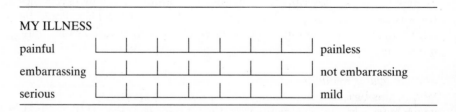

MY ILLNESS

painful   painless

embarrassing   not embarrassing

serious   mild

Fig. 4.6 The semantic differential scale.

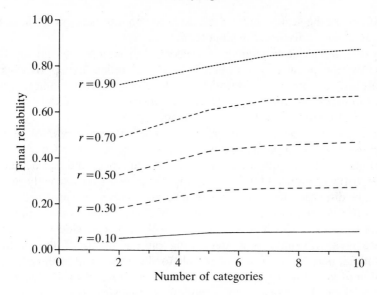

Fig. 4.7 The effect of the number of scale categories on reliability.

categories are used. Nishisato and Torii (1970) studied this empirically by generating distributions of two variables with known correlations, ranging from 0.1 to 0.9 in steps of 0.2. They then rounded off the numbers as if they were creating a scale of a particular number of steps. For example, if the original numbers fell in the range from 1.000 to 10.000, a two-point scale was created by calling any number less than 5.000 a 0, and any number greater than or equal to 5.000 a 1. A ten-point scale was created by rounding off up to the decimal point, resulting in discrete values ranging from 1 to 10. The final step in this simulation was to recalculate the correlation using the rounded numbers. Since the rounding process resulted in the loss of precision, this should have the effect of reducing the correlation between the sets of numbers. The original correlation corresponds to the test–retest reliability of the original data, and the recalculated correlation, using the rounded-off numbers is equivalent to the reliability which would result from a scale with 2, 5 or 10 boxes, with everything else held constant.

As can be seen from Figure 4.7, the loss in reliability for 7 and 10 categories is quite small. However, the use of five categories reduces the reliability by about 12 per cent, and the use of only two categories results in an average reduction of the reliability coefficient of 35 per cent. These results were confirmed by other studies, and suggest that the minimum number of categories used by raters should be in the region of five to seven. Of course, a common problem of ratings is that raters seldom use the extreme

positions on the scale, and this should be taken into account when designing the scale, as discussed in Chapter 6.

2. *Is there a maximum number of categories?* From a purely statistical perspective, the answer is 'no', since the actual reliability approaches the
theoretical maximum asymptotically. However, there is some evidence
that too many categories may adversely affect ratings (Conklin 1923), and
10 to 15 categories is probably a reasonable upper limit.

3. *Should there be an even or odd number of categories?* Where the
response scale is unipolar, that is to say, scale values range from zero to a
maximum, then the question is of little consequence, and can be decided
on stylistic grounds. However for bipolar scales (like strongly agree—
strongly disagree) the provision of an odd number of categories allows
raters the choice of expressing no opinion. Conversely, an even number of
boxes forces the raters to commit themselves to one side or the other.
There is no absolute rule; depending on the needs of the particular
research it may or may not be desirable to allow a neutral position.

4. *Should the order of successive question responses change?* Some scales
reverse the order of responses at random, so that successive questions may
have response categories which go from low to high or high to low, in order
to avoid 'yea-saying' bias (discussed in Chapter 6). The dilemma is that a
careless subject may not notice the change, resulting in almost totally uninterpretable responses. Of course, with reversed order, the researcher will
know that the responses are uninterpretable due to carelessness, whereas if
order is not reversed the subject looks consistent whether or not he paid
attention to individual questions.

5. *Can it be assumed that the data are interval?* As we indicated earlier, one
issue regarding the use of rating scales is that they are, strictly speaking, on
an ordinal level of measurement. Although responses are routinely
assigned numerical values, so that 'strongly agree' becomes a 7 and
'strongly disagree' becomes a 1, we really have no guarantee that the true
distance between successive categories is the same; i.e. that the distance
between 'strongly agree' and 'agree' is really the same as the distance
between 'strongly disagree' and 'disagree'. The matter is of more than
theoretical interest, since the statistical methods which are used to analyse
the data, such as analysis of variance, rest on this assumption of equality of
distance. Considerable debate has surrounded the dangers inherent in the
assumption of interval properties. The arguments range from the extreme
position that the numbers themselves are interval (e.g. 1,2, . . . ,7) and can
be manipulated as interval-level data regardless of their relationship to the
underlying property being assessed (Gaito 1982) to the opposite view that
the numbers must be demonstrated to have a linear relationship with the
underlying property before interval-level measurement can be assumed
(Townsend and Ashby 1984). The debate shows no sign of resolution.

Nevertheless, from a pragmatic viewpoint, it appears that under most circumstances, unless the distribution of scores is severely skewed, one can analyse data from rating scales as if they were interval without introducing severe bias.

Critique of direct estimation methods

Direct estimation methods, in various forms, are pervasive in research involving subjective judgements. They are relatively easy to design, require little pre-testing in contrast to the comparative methods described next, and are easily understood by subjects. Nevertheless, the ease of design and administration is both an asset and a liability: because the intent of questions framed on a rating scale is often obvious to both researcher and respondent, bias in response can result. The issue of bias is covered in more detail in Chapter 6; but we mention some problems briefly here. One bias of rating scales is the *halo effect*; since items are frequently ordered in a single column on a page it is possible to rapidly rate all items on the basis of a global impression, paying little attention to the individual categories. People also rarely commit themselves to the extreme categories on the scale, effectively reducing the precision of measurement. Finally, it is common in ratings of other people, staff or students, to have a strong positive skew, so that the average individual is rated well above average, again sacrificing precision.

In choosing among specific methods, the scaling methods we have described differ for historical rather than substantive reasons, and it is easy to find examples which have features of more than one approach. The important point is to follow the general guidelines: specific descriptors, seven or more steps, and so forth, rather than becoming preoccupied with choosing among alternatives.

Comparative methods

Although rating scales have a number of advantages—simplicity, ease and speed of completion—there are occasions where their simplicity would be a deterrent to acquiring useful data. For example, in a study of predictors of child abuse (Shearman *et al.* 1983), one scale questioned parents on the ways they handled irritating child behaviours. A number of infant behaviours were presented, and parents were to specify how they dealt with each problem. Casting this scale into a rating format (which was not done) might result in items like those in Figure 4.8.

The ordered nature of the response scale would make it unlikely that parents would place any marks to the left of the neutral position. Instead, we would like the respondent to simply indicate her likely action, or select it from a list. If we could then assign a value to each behaviour, we could

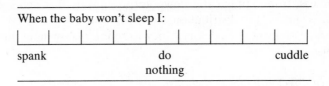

Fig. 4.8 Likert scaling of a question about child abuse.

generate a score for the respondent based on the sum of the assigned values.

The approach which was used was one of a class of *comparative* methods, called the *paired-comparison* technique, whereby respondents were simply asked to indicate which behaviour—'punish', 'cuddle', 'hit', 'ignore', 'put in room'—they were likely to do in a particular circumstance. These individual responses were assigned a numerical value in advance on the basis of a survey of a group of experts (in this case day-care workers), who had been asked to compare each parental response to a situation to all other possible responses, and select the most appropriate response for each of these pairwise comparisons.

The comparative methods also address a general problem with all rating scales, the ordinal nature of the scale. Comparative methods circumvent the difficulty by directly scaling the value of each description before obtaining responses, to ensure that the response values are on an interval scale.

There are three comparative methods commonly used in the literature: *Thurstone's method* of equal-appearing intervals, *Guttman scaling*, and the *paired-comparison* technique. Each is discussed below.

Thurstone's method of equal-appearing intervals
The method begins with the selection of 100–200 statements relevant to the topic about which attitudes are to be assessed. Following the usual approaches to item generation, these statements are edited to be short and to the point. Each statement is then typed on a separate card, and a number of judges are asked to sort them into a single pile from the lowest or least desirable to highest. Extreme anchor statements, at the opposite ends of the scale, may be provided. Following the completion of this task by a large number of judges, the median rank of each statement is computed, which then becomes the scale value for each statement.

As an example, if we were assessing attitude to doctors, we might assemble a large number of statements like 'I will always do anything my doctor prescribes', 'I think doctors are overpaid', and 'Most doctors are aware of their patients' feelings'. Suppose we gave these statements to nine judges (actually, many more would be necessary for stable estimates) and the statement 'I think nurses provide as good care as doctors' was ranked respectively by the nine judges 17, 18, 23, 25, 26, 27, 28, 31, and 35, of 100 statements. The median rank of this statement is the rank of the fifth person, in this case 26, so this would be the value assigned to the statement.

The next step in the procedure is to select a limited number of statements, about 25 in number, in such a manner that the intervals between successive items are about equal and they span the entire range of values. These items then comprise the actual scale.

Finally, in applying the scale to an individual, the respondent is asked to indicate which statements apply to him/her. The respondents' score is then calculated as the average score of items selected.

Paired comparison technique
The paired-comparison method is directed at similar goals, and uses a similar approach to the Thurstone method. In both methods, the initial step is to calibrate a limited set of items so that they can be placed on an interval scale. Subjects' responses to these items are then used in developing a score by simply summing or averaging the calibration weights of those items endorsed by a subject.

Where the two methods differ is in their approach to calibration. Thurstone scaling begins with a large number of items, and asks people to judge each item against all others by explicitly ranking the items. By contrast, the paired-comparison method, as the name implies, asks judges to explicitly compare each item one at a time to each of the remaining items, and simply judge which of the two has more of the property under study. Considering the example which began this chapter, our child care workers would be asked to indicate the more desirable parental behaviour in pairwise fashion as follows:

punish—spank
punish—cuddle
punish—ignore
spank—cuddle
spank—ignore
cuddle—ignore

In actual practice, a larger sample of parental behaviours would be used, order from right to left would be randomized, and the order of presentation of the cards would be randomized.

If such a list of choices were given to a series of ten judges, the data would be then displayed as in Table 4.1, indicating the proportion of times each alternative was chosen over each other option.

Reading down the first column, the table shows, for example that 'punish' was chosen over 'spank' by 40 per cent of the subjects. Note that the diagonal entries are assumed equal to 0.50, i.e. 'punish' is selected over

Table 4.1 *Probability of selecting each behaviour over others*

Behaviour	1 Punish	2 Spank	3 Ignore	4 Cuddle
1. Punish	0.50	0.60	0.70	0.90
2. Spank	0.40	0.50	0.70	0.80
3. Ignore	0.30	0.30	0.50	0.70
4. Cuddle	0.10	0.20	0.30	0.50

'punish' 50 per cent of the time; also, the top right values are the 'mirror image' of those in the bottom left.

The next step is to use the property of the normal curve to convert this table to z-values. This bit of sleight-of-hand is best illustrated by reference to Figure 4.9, which shows the 40 per cent point on a normal curve; that is, the point on the curve where 40 per cent of the distribution falls to the left. If the mean of the curve is set to zero, and the standard deviation to 1, this occurs at a value of -0.26. As a result, the probability value of 0.40 is

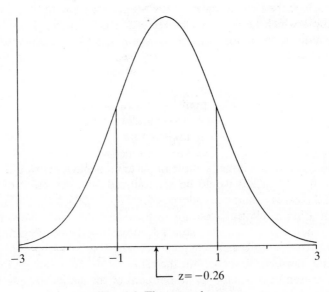

Fig. 4.9 The normal curve.

replaced by a z-value of -0.26. In practice, these values are determined by consulting a table of the normal curve in any statistical text. The resulting values are shown in Table 4.2.

The z scores for each column are then summed and averaged, yielding the z score equivalent to the average probability of each item being selected over all other items. The resulting z score for 'punish' now becomes -2.39, and for 'cuddle' it is $+2.66$. The range of negative and positive numbers is a bit awkward, so a constant is often added to all the values to avoid negative weights. These weights can be assumed to have interval properties.

All this manipulation is directed to the assignment of weights to each option. To use these weights for scoring a subject is straightforward; the score is simply the weight assigned to the option selected by the subject. If the questionnaire is designed in such a way that a subject may endorse mul-tiple-response options, for example by responding to various infant behav-iours like crying, not going to sleep, refusing to eat, the weights for all responses can be added or averaged since they are interval level measure-ments.

The Guttman method
The Guttman method begins, as does the Thurstone method, with a large sample of items. However, this is reduced by judgement of the investigator to a relatively small sample of 10–20 items which are thought to span the range of the attitude or behaviour assessed. As we shall see, in Guttman scaling, it is crucial that the items address only a single underlying attri-bute, since an individual score arises from the accumulated performance on all items.

These items are then administered directly to a sample of subjects, who are asked to endorse those items applicable to them. Unlike the alternative

Table 4.2 *z-values of the probabilities*

Behaviour	1	2	3	4
1. Punish	0.00	0.26	0.53	1.28
2. Spank	−0.26	0.00	0.53	0.85
3. Ignore	−0.85	−0.85	0.00	0.53
4. Cuddle	−1.28	−0.85	−0.53	0.00
Total z	−2.39	−1.44	+0.53	+2.66
Average z	−0.59	−0.36	+0.13	+0.66

Table 4.3   *Guttman scaling*

I am able to:	Subject
	A B C D E
Walk across the room	1 1 1 1 1
Climb the stairs	1 1 1 1 0
Walk one block outdoors	1 1 0 0 0
Walk more than one mile	1 0 0 0 0

methods discussed in this section, there is no separate calibration step. The items are then tentatively ranked according to increasing amount of the attribute assessed, and responses are displayed in a subject-by-item matrix, with 1's indicating those items endorsed by a subject and 0's indicating the remaining items.

As an example, suppose we were assessing function of the lower limbs in a sample of people with osteo-arthritis. A display of the responses of five subjects to the following four items might resemble Table 4.3.

On this scale, subject A is assigned a score of 4, 3 for subject B, 2 for C and D, and 1 for E. The example is an idealized version since no 'reversals' occurred, in which some subjects endorsed a lower-ranked statement. In fact, it is very difficult to construct a scale with Guttman properties, since any departure from unidimensionality, or any random variation, will result in a disruption of the strict ordering implied by the method. Further, although the other methods considered in this section are explicit attempts to ensure interval-level responses, the Guttman scale, which demands only ordered categories, is highly unlikely to meet the assumption of interval scaling.

Guttman scaling is best suited to behaviours which are developmentally determined (e.g., crawling, standing, walking, running), where mastery of one behaviour virtually guarantees mastery of lower-order behaviours. Thus it is useful in assessing development in children, decline due to progressively deteriorating disease, functional ability, and the like. It is *not* appropriate in assessing the kind of loss in function due to focal lesions that arises in stroke patients, where impairment of some function may be unrelated to impairment of other functions.

Guttman scaling is also the basis of *latent-trait theory* (discussed in Chapter 12), which has emerged as a very powerful scaling method, and begins with a similar assumption of ordering of item difficulty and candidate ability. However, in contrast to Guttman scaling, latent-trait scaling explicitly assigns values to both items and subjects on an interval scale, and also deals successfully with the random processes which might result in departures from strict ordering demanded by the Guttman scale.

Critique of comparative methods

It is clear that any of the three comparative methods we have described requires considerably more time for development than any of the direct scaling methods. Nevertheless, this investment may be worthwhile under two circumstances. If it is desirable to disguise the ordinal property of the responses, as in the child abuse example, then the additional resources may be well spent. Secondly, the Thurstone and paired-comparison methods guarantee interval-level measurement, which may be important in some applications, particularly when there are relatively few items in the scale.

With regard to choice among the methods, as we have indicated, the Guttman method has several disadvantages in comparison to other methods. It is difficult to select items with Guttman properties, and the scale has only ordinal properties. The choice between Thurstone and paired-comparison is more difficult. However, the Thurstone method is more practical when there are a large number of items desired in the scale, since the number of comparisons needed in the paired-comparison technique is roughly proportional to the square of the number of items.

Econometric methods

The final class of scaling methods we will consider has its roots in a different discipline, economics, and has become increasingly popular in the medical literature in applications ranging from clinical trials to decision analysis. The problem for which these methods were devised involves assigning a numerical value to various health states. This arises in economics and health in the course of conducting cost/benefit studies, where it becomes necessary to scale benefits along a numerical scale so that cost/benefit ratios can be determined.

For example, consider a clinical trial comparing medical management of angina to coronary bypass surgery. Surgery offers a potential benefit in quality of life, but the tradeoff is the finite possibility that the patient may not survive the operation or immediate post-operative period. How, then, does one make a rational choice between the two alternatives?

The first approach to the problem was developed in the 1950s, and is called the *Von Neumann–Morgenstern standard gamble* (1953). The subject is asked to consider the following scenario:

'You have been suffering from 'angina' for several years. As a result of your illness, you experience severe chest pain after even minor physical exertion such as climbing stairs, or walking one block in cold weather. You have been forced to quit your job, and spend most days at home watching TV. Imagine that you are offered a possibility of an operation that will result in complete recovery from your illness. However, the operation carries some risk. Specifically, there is a probability '*p*' that you will die during the course of the operation. How large must '*p*' be before you will decline the operation and choose to remain in your present state?'

Clearly, the closer the present state is to perfect health, the smaller the risk of death one would be willing to entertain. Having obtained an estimate of '*p*' from subjects, the value of the present state can be directly converted to a 0–1 scale by simply subtracting '*p*' from 1, so that a tolerable risk of 1 per cent results in a value (called a 'utility') of 0.99 for the present state, and a risk of 50 per cent results in a utility of 0.50.

One difficulty with the 'standard gamble' is that few people, aside from statisticians and professional gamblers, are accustomed to dealing in probabilities. In order to deal with this problem, a number of devices are used to simplify the task. Subjects may be offered specific probabilities; e.g., 10 per cent chance of perioperative death, and 90 per cent chance of complete recovery, until they reach a point of indifference between the two alternatives. Visual aids, such as 'probability wheels', have also been used.

This difficulty in handling probabilities led to the development of an alternative method, called the *time tradeoff technique* (Torrance *et al.* 1972), which avoids the use of probabilities. One begins by estimating the likely remaining years of life for a healthy subject, using actuarial tables; i.e. if the patient is 30 years old we could estimate that he has about 40 years remaining. The previous question would then be rephrased as follows:
'Imagine living the remainder of your natural lifespan (40 years) in your present state. Contrast this with the alternative that you can return to perfect health for fewer years. How many years would you sacrifice if you could have perfect health?'

In practice, the respondent is presented with the alternatives of 40 years in her present state versus 0 years of complete health. The upper limit is decreased, and the lower limit increased, until a point of indifference is reached. The more years a subject is willing to sacrifice in exchange for a return to perfect health, presumably the worse he perceives his present health. The response (call it Y) can be converted to a scaled utility by the simple formula

$$U = (40 - Y)/40.$$

A thorough example of the application of this method in a clinical trial of support for relatives of demented elderly is given in Mohide *et al.* (1988).

Critique of econometric methods
We have presented the two methods as a means to measure individual health states. Although they are limited to the measurement of health

states, they have been used both with real patients and with normal, healthy individuals imagining themselves to be ill.

The methods are quite difficult to administer and require a trained interviewer, so it remains to see whether they possess advantages over simpler techniques. One straightforward alternative would be a direct estimation of health state, using an adjectival or visual analogue scale. Torrance (1976) has shown that the time tradeoff and standard gamble methods yield similar results, which differed from the direct estimation method, suggesting that these methods may indeed be a more accurate reflection of the underlying state.

However, the methods are based on the notion that people make rational choices under conditions of uncertainty. There is an accumulation of evidence, reviewed in Chapter 6, which suggests that responses on rating scales can be influenced by a variety of extraneous factors. The methods reviewed in this section are no more immune to seemingly irrational behaviour, as reviewed by Llewellyn-Thomas and Sutherland (1986). As one example, framing a question in terms of 40 per cent survival instead of 60 per cent mortality will result in a shift of values. The problem addressed by the econometric methods assumed that context-free values could be elicited. It seems abundantly clear that such 'value-free' values are illusory, and a deeper understanding of the psychological variables which influence decisions and choices is necessary. Moreover, it appears that real patients assign higher (more positive) utilities to states of ill health than do normals imagining themselves in that state, casting doubt on the analogue studies. Last, the lower anchor is usually assumed to be death. There has been little work to examine conditions which some people (for example, Richard Dreyfuss in the movie *Whose Life Is It Anyway*) see as worse than death.

References

Aitken, R. C. B. (1969). A growing edge of measurement of feelings. *Proceedings of the Royal Society of Medicine*, **62**, 989–92.

Conklin, E.S. (1923) *The scale of value method for studies in genetic psychology*. University of Oregon Publications, Eugene.

Downie W. W., Leatham, P. A., Rhind, V. M., Wright, V., Branco, J. A., and Anderson, J. A. (1978). Studies with pain rating scales. *Annals of Rheumatic Diseases*, **37**, 378–81.

Gaito, J. (1982). Measurement scales and statistics: Resurgence of an old misconception. *Psychological Bulletin*, **87**, 564–7.

Guilford, J. P. (1954). *Psychometric methods*. McGraw-Hill, New York.

Huskisson, E. C. (1974). Measurement of pain. *Lancet*, **ii**, 1127–31.

Likert, R. A. (1952). A technique for the development of attitude scales. *Educational and Psychological Measurement*, **12**, 313–15.

Llewellyn-Thomas, H., and Sutherland, H. (1986). Procedures for value assessment. In *Recent Advances in nursing: Research methodology*. (ed. M. Calhoun) Churchill-Livingstone, London.

Mohide, E. A., Torrance, G. W., Streiner, D. L., Pringle, D. M., and Gilbert, J. R. (1988). Measuring the well-being of family caregivers using the time tradeoff technique. *Journal of Clinical Epidemiology*, **41**, 475–82.

Nishisato, N., and Torii, Y. (1970). Effects of categorizing continuous normal distributions on the product-moment correlation. *Japanese Psychological Research*, **13**, 45–9.

Osgood, C., Suci, G., and Tannenbaum, P. (1957). *The measurement of feeling*. University of Illinois Press, Urbana.

Scott, P. J., and Huskisson, E. C. (1978). Measurement of functional capacity with visual analogue scales. *Rheumatology and Rehabilitation*, **16**, 257–9.

Scott, P. J., and Huskisson, E. C. (1979). Accuracy of subjective measurements made with and without previous scores: An important source of error in serial measurement of subjective states. *Annals of Rheumatic Diseases*, **38**, 558–9.

Shearman, J. K., Evans, C. E. E., Boyle, M. H., Cuddy, L. J., and Norman, G. R. (1983). Maternal and infant characteristics in abuse: A case control study. *Journal of Family Practice*, **16**, 289–93.

Torrance, G. (1976). Social preferences for health states: An empirical evaluation of three measurement techniques. *Socio-Economic Planning Sciences*, **10**, 129–36.

Torrance, G., Thomas, W. H., and Sackett, D. L. (1972). A utility maximization model for evaluation of health care programs. *Health Services Research*, **7**, 118–33.

Townsend, J. T., and Ashby, F. G. (1984). Measurement scales and statistics: The misconception misconceived. *Psychological Bulletin*, **96**, 394–401.

Von Neumann, J., and Morgenstern, O. (1953). *The theory of games and economic behavior*. Wiley, New York.

5

Selecting the items

In previous chapters, we have discussed how to develop items which would be included in the new scale. Obviously, not all of the items will work as intended; some may be confusing to the respondent, some may not tell us what we thought they would, and so on. Here we examine various criteria used in determining which ones to retain and which to discard.

Interpretability

The first criterion for selecting items is to eliminate any which are ambiguous or incomprehensible. Problems can arise from any one of a number of sources: the words are too difficult; they contain jargon terms which are used only by certain groups of people, such as health professionals; or they are 'double-barrelled'.

Reading level

Except for scales which are aimed at a selected group whose educational level is known, the usual rule of thumb is that the scale should not require reading skills beyond that of a 12 year old. This may seem unduly low, but many people who are high-school graduates are unable to comprehend material much above this level. Many ways have been proposed to assess the reading level required to understand written material. Some methods, like the 'cloze' technique (Taylor 1957), eliminate every nth word to see at what point meaning disappears; the easier the material, the more words can be removed and accurately 'filled in' by the reader. Other methods are based on the number of syllables in each word or the number of words in each sentence (e.g. Flesch 1948; Fry 1968). However, these procedures can be laborious and time-consuming, and others may require up to 300 words of text (e.g. McLaughlin 1969). These are usually inappropriate for scales or questionnaires, where each item is an independent passage, and meaning may depend on one key word.

Another method is to use a list of words which are comprehensible at each grade level (e.g. Dale and Eichholz 1960). While it may be impractical (and even unnecessary) to check every word in the scale, those which appear to be difficult can be checked. Even glancing through one of these books can give the scale developer a rough idea of the complexity of Grade 6 words. Approaching the problem from the other direction, Payne (1954) compiled a very useful list of 1000 common words, indicating whether each was unambiguous, problematic, or had multiple meanings.

Perhaps the most practical technique is to pretest the instrument on a group of people comparable to those who will be the ultimate targets. These people are asked to read each item, and indicate if they understand it; they are not asked to actually respond to the questions. The instrument developer can probe if he or she is unsure whether the person actually understood all of the words used in the item. A common mistake is to use one's colleagues or other convenient samples which may bear little resemblance to the final user population.

Ambiguity

This same method is often used to determine if the items are ambiguous or poorly worded. Even a seemingly straightforward item such as 'I like my mother', can pose a problem if the respondent's mother is dead. Some people answer by assuming that the sentence can also be read in the past tense, while others may simply say 'no', reflecting the fact that they can't like her now. On a questionnaire designed to assess patients' attitudes to their recent hospitalization, one item asked about information given to the patient by various people. A stem read 'I understand what was told to me by:', followed by a list of different health care professionals, with room to check either 'yes' or 'no'. Here, a 'no' response opposite 'Social Worker', for instance, could indicate
- that the patient did not understand what the social worker said,
- that she never saw a social worker, or
- that she does not remember whether she saw the social worker or not.

While these latter two possibilities were not what the test developer intended, the ambiguity of the question and the response scheme forced the subject to respond with an ambiguous answer.

Ambiguity can also arise by the vagueness of the response alternatives. The answer to the question, 'Have you seen your doctor recently' depends on the subject's interpretation of 'recently'. One person may feel that it refers to the previous week, another to the past month, and a third person may believe it covers the previous year. Even if we rephrase the question to use a seemingly more specific term, ambiguity can remain. 'Have you seen your doctor during the past year?' can mean
- during the last 12 months, more or less,
- since this date one year ago, or
- since 1 January of this year.

If a specific time frame (or any another variable) is called for, it should be spelled out explicitly. Questionnaire developers vastly overestimate people's ability to recall past events. The evidence is that people have difficulty remembering episodes of illness even over short periods of time, and especially when they did not receive medical help (Allen *et al.* 1954). Thus, the replies to questions like, 'Compared to how you felt a year ago . . . ' should be viewed with some degree of scepticism.

Double-barrelled question

A 'double-barrelled' item is one that asks two or more questions at the same time, each of which can be answered differently. These are unfortunately quite common in questionnaires probing for physical or psychological symptoms, such as 'My eyes are red and teary'. How should one answer if one's eyes are red but not teary or teary but not red? Since some people will say 'yes' only if both parts are true, while others will respond this way if either symptom was present, the final result may not reflect the actual state of affairs. Pre-testing on a large group, where it is likely that some people will fall into these grey areas, can reduce the risk of these types of items occurring.

Jargon

Jargon terms can slip into a scale or questionnaire quite insidiously. Since we use a technical vocabulary on a daily basis, and these terms are fully understood by our colleagues, it is easy to overlook the fact that these words are not part of the everyday vocabulary of others, or may have very different connotations. Terms like 'lesion', 'care-giver', or 'range of motion' may not be ones which the average person understands. Even more troublesome are words which *are* understood, but in a manner different from what the scale developer intended. 'Hypertension', for example, means 'being very tense' to some people; and asking some what colour their stool is may elicit the rsponse that the problem is with their gut, not their furniture. Again, pre-testing is desirable, with the interviewer asking the people not whether they had the complaint, but rather what they think the term means.

Value-laden words

A final factor affecting the interpretation of the question is the use of value-laden terms. Items such as 'Do you often go to your doctor with trivial problems?' or 'Do physicians make too much money?' may prejudice the respondents, leading them to answer as much to the tenor of the question as to its content. (Both items also contain ambiguous terms, such as 'often', 'trivial', and 'too much'.) Naturally, such value-laden terms should be avoided.

Positive and negative wording

As a general rule, scale developers should avoid negatively worded items; that is, items which use words such as 'not', 'rarely', or 'never', or which have words with negative prefixes (e.g., in-, im-, or un-). Such items tend to have lower validity coefficients than positively worded ones (Holden *et al*. 1985; Schriesheim and Hill 1981). It would be better to have an item which states 'I feel ill most of the time', for example, rather than 'I rarely feel well'.

Length of items

Items on scales should be as short as possible, although not so short that comprehensibility is lost. Item validity coefficients tend to fall as the number of letters in the item increases. Holden *et al*. (1985) found that, on average, items with 70–80 letters had validity coefficients under 0.10, while items containing 10–20 characters had coefficients almost four times higher.

Rechecking

Even after all of the items have passed these checks and have been incorporated into the scale, it is worthwhile to check them over informally every year or so to see if any terms may have taken on new meanings. For example, liking to go to 'gay parties' has a very different connotation now than it did some years ago, when to most people the word 'gay' had no association with homosexuality.

Face validity

One issue that must be decided before the items are written or selected is whether or not they should have *face validity*. That is, do the items appear on the surface to be measuring what they actually are? As is often the case, there are two schools of thought on this issue, and the 'correct' answer often depends on the purpose that the measure will be used for.

Those who argue for face validity state, quite convincingly, that it increases the acceptance of the instrument by those who will ultimately use it. If the item appears irrelevant, then the respondent may very well object to it or omit it, irrespective of its possibly superb psychometric properties. For example, it is commonly believed that some psychiatric patients manifest increased religiosity, especially during the acute phase of their illness. Capitalizing on this fact, the MMPI contains a few items tapping into this domain. Despite the fact that these items are psychometrically quite good, it has opened the test to much (perhaps unnecessary) criticism for delving into seemingly irrelevant, private matters.

On the other hand, it may be necessary in some circumstances to disguise the true nature of the question, lest the respondents try to 'fake' their answers, an issue we will return to in greater detail in Chapter 6. For example, patients may want to appear worse than they actually are in order to ensure that they will receive help; or better than they really feel in order to please the doctor. This is easy to do if the items have face validity—that is, their meaning and relevance are self-evident—and much harder if they do not. Thus, the ultimate decision depends on the nature and purpose of the instrument.

Frequency of endorsement and discrimination

After the scale has been pretested for readability and absence of ambiguity, it is then given to a large group of subjects to test for other attributes, including the endorsement frequency. (The meaning of 'large' is variable, but usually 50 subjects would be an absolute minimum.) The frequency of endorsement is simply the proportion of people (p) who give each response alternative to an item. For dichotomous items, this reduces to simply the proportion saying 'yes' (or, conversely, 'no'). A multiple-choice item has a number of 'frequencies of endorsement;' the proportion choosing alternative A, one for alternative B, and so forth.

In achievement tests, the frequency of endorsement is a function of the *difficulty* of the item, with a specific response alternative reflecting the correct answer. For personality measures, the frequency of endorsement is the 'popularity' of that item; the proportion of people who choose the alternative which indicates more of the trait, attitude, or behaviour (Allen and Yen 1979).

Usually, items where one alternative has a very high (or low) endorsement rates are eliminated. If p is over 0.95 (or under 0.05), then most people are responding in the same direction or with the same alternative. Since we can predict what the answer will be with greater than 95 per cent accuracy, we learn very little by knowing how a person actually responded. Such questions do not improve a scale's psychometric properties, and may actually detract from them while making the test longer. In practice, only items with endorsement rates between 0.20 and 0.80 are used.

There are some scales, though, which are deliberately made up of items with a high endorsement frequency. This is the case where there may be some question regarding the subject's ability or willingness to answer honestly. A person may not read the item accurately because of factors such as illiteracy, retardation, or difficulties in concentration; or may not answer honestly because of an attempt to 'fake' a response for some reason. Some tests, like the MMPI or the *Personality Research Form* (Jackson 1984), have special scales to detect these biases, comprised of a heterogeneous group of items which have only one thing in common: an endorsement frequency of 90–95 per cent. To get rates this high, the questions have to be either quite bizarre (e.g., 'I have never touched money') or extremely banal ('I eat most days'). A significant number of questions answered in the 'wrong' direction is a flag that the person was not reading the items carefully and responding as would most people. This may temper the interpretation given to other scales that the person completes.

Another index of the utility of an item, closely related to endorsement frequency, is its *discrimination* ability. This tells us if a person who has a high total score is more likely to have endorsed the item; conversely, if the item discriminates between those who score high (and supposedly have more of the trait) and those who score low. It is related to endorsement frequency in that, from a psychometric viewpoint, items which discriminate best among people have values of p near the cut-point of the scale. It differs in that it looks at the item in relation to all of the other items on the scale, not just in isolation.

A simple item discrimination index is given by the formula

$$d_i = \frac{U_i - L_i}{n_i},$$

where U_i is the number of people above the median who score positive on item i, L_i is the number of people below the median who score positive on item i, and n_i is the number of people above (or below) the median.

Homogeneity of the items

In most situations, whenever we are measuring a trait, behaviour, or symptom, we want the scale to be homogeneous. That is, all of the items should be tapping different aspects of the same attribute, and not different parts of different traits. (Later in this chapter we deal with the situation where we want the test to measure a variety of characteristics.) For example, if we were measuring the problem-solving ability of medical students, then each item should relate to problem solving. This has two implications:

- the items should be moderately correlated with each other, and
- each should correlate with the total scale score.

Indeed, these two factors form the basis of the various tests of homogeneity or 'internal consistency' of the scale.

Before the mechanics of measuring internal consistency are discussed, some rationale and background are in order. In almost all areas we measure, a simple summing of the scores over the individual items is the most sensible index; this point will be returned to in Chapter 7. However, this 'linear model' approach (Nunnally 1970) works only if all items are measuring the same trait. If the items were measuring different attributes, it would not be logical to add them up to form one total score. On the other hand, if one item were highly correlated with a second one, then the latter question would add little additional information. Hence there is a need to derive some quantitative measure of the degree to which items are related to each other; i.e., the degree of 'homogeneity' of the scale.

Current thinking in test development holds that there should be a moderate correlation among the items in a scale. If the items were chosen without regard for homogeneity, then the resulting scale could possibly end up tapping a number of traits. If the correlations were too high, there would be much redundancy, and a possible loss of content validity.

It should be noted that this position of taking homogeneity into account, which is most closely identified with Jackson (1970) and Nunnally (1970), is not shared by all psychometricians. Another school of thought is that internal consistency and face validity make sense if the primary aim is to *describe* a trait, behaviour, or disorder, but not necessarily if the goal is to *discriminate* people who have an attribute from those who do not. That is, if we are trying to measure the degree of depression, for example, the scale should *appear* to be measuring it and all of the items should relate to this in a coherent manner. On the other hand, if our aim is to *discriminate* depressed patients from other groups, then it is sufficient to choose items which are answered differently by the depressed group, irrespective of their content. This in fact was the method used in constructing the MMPI, one of the most famous paper-and-pencil questionnaires for psychological assessment. An item was included in the Depression Scale (*D*) based on the criterion that depressed patients responded to it in one way significantly more often than did non-depressed people, and without regard for the correlation among the individual items. As a result, the *D* scale has some items which seem to be related to depression, but also many other items which do not. On the other hand, the more recent CES-D (Radloff 1977), which measures depressive symptomatology without diagnosing depression, was constructed following the philosophy of high internal consistency, and its items all appear to be tapping into this domain. If a trend can be detected, it is toward scales that are more grounded in theory and are more internally consistent, and away from the empiricism that led to the MMPI.

One last comment is in order before discussing the techniques of item selection. Many inventories, especially those in the realms of psychology and psychiatry, are multidimensional; that is, they are comprised of a number of different scales, with the items intermixed in a random manner. Measures of homogeneity should be applied to the individual scales, as it does not make sense to talk of homogeneity across different subscales.

Item–total correlation

One of the oldest, albeit still widely used, methods for checking the homogeneity of the scale is the *item–total correlation*. As the name implies, it is the correlation of the individual item with the scale total *omitting that item*. If we did not remove the item from the total score, the correlation would be artificially inflated, since it would be based in part on the item correlated with itself. The item can be eliminated in one of two ways; physically or statistically. We can physically remove the item by not including it when calculating the total score. So, for a five-item scale, Item 1 would be correlated with the sum of Items 2–5; Item 2 with the sum of 1 and 3–5; and so on. One problem with this approach is that, for a k-item scale, we have to calculate the total score k times; not a difficult problem, but a laborious one, especially if a computer program to do this is not readily available.

The second method is statistical; the item's contribution to the total score is removed using the formula given by Nunnally (1978):

$$r_{i(t-1)} = \frac{r_{it}\,\sigma_t - \sigma_i}{\sqrt{(\sigma_i^2 + \sigma_t^2 - 2\sigma_i\,\sigma_t\,r_{it})}},$$

where $r_{i(t-1)}$ is the correlation of item i with the total, removing the effect of item i, r_{it} is the correlation of item i with the total score, σ_i is the standard deviation of item i; and σ_t is the standard deviation of the total scores.

The usual rule of thumb is that an item should correlate with the total score above 0.20. Items with lower correlations should be discarded (Kline 1986).

In almost all instances, the best coefficient to use is the *Pearson product-moment correlation* (Nunnally 1970). If the items are dichotomous, then the usually recommended point-biserial correlation yields identical results; if there are more than two response alternatives, the product-moment correlation is robust enough to produce relatively accurate results, even if the data are not normally distributed (see for example Havlicek and Peterson 1977).

Split-half reliability

Another approach to testing the homogeneity of a scale is called *split-half reliability*. Here, the items are randomly divided into two sub-scales, which are then correlated with each other. This is also referred to as 'odd—even' reliability, since the easiest split is to put all odd-numbered items in one half and even-numbered ones in the other. If the scale is internally consistent, then the two halves should correlate highly.

One problem is that the resulting correlation is an underestimate of the true reliability of the scale, since the reliability of a scale is directly proportional to the number of items in it. Since the sub-scales being correlated are only half the length of the version that will be used in practice, the resulting correlation will be too low. The Spearman–Brown 'prophesy' formula is used to correct for this occurrence. The equation for this is

$$r_{SB} = \frac{kr}{1 + (k-1)r},$$

wnere k is the factor by which the scale is to be increased or decreased, and r is the original correlation.

In this case, we want to see the result when there are twice the number of items, so k is set at 2. For example, if we found that splitting a 40-item scale in half yields a correlation of 0.50, we would substitute into the equation as follows:

$$r_{SB} = \frac{2 \times 0.50}{1 + (2-1) \times 0.50}.$$

Thus, the estimate of the split-half reliability of this scale would be 0.67.

Since there are many ways to divide a test into two parts, there are in fact many possible split-half reliabilities; a 10-item test can be divided 126 ways, a 12-item test 462 different ways, and so on. (These numbers represent the combination of n items taken $n/2$ at a time. This is then divided by 2, since (assuming a six-item scale) items 1, 2, and 3 in the first half and 4, 5, and 6 in the second is the same as 4, 5, and 6 in the first part and the remaining items in the second.) These reliability coefficients may differ quite considerably from one split to another.

There are two situations where we should *not* divide a test randomly; highly timed achievement tests, and tests with serially related items. In the former case, where the major emphasis is on how quickly a person can work, most of the items are fairly easy, and failure is due to not reaching that question before the time limit. Thus, the answers up to the timed cut-off will almost all be correct, and those after it all incorrect. Any split-half reliability will yield a very high value, only marginally lower than 1.0.

With related or 'chained' items, failure on the second item could occur in two ways: not being able to answer it correctly; or being able to do it, but getting it wrong, because of an erroneous response to the previous item. For example, assume that the two (relatively simple) items were:

A. The organ for pumping blood is:
   1. The pineal gland
   2. The heart
   3. The stomach
B. It is located in:
   1. The chest
   2. The gut
   3. The skull

If the answer to A were correct, then a wrong response to B would indicate that the person did not know where the heart is located. However, if A and B were wrong, then the person *may* have known that the heart is located in the chest, but went astray in believing that blood is pumped by the pineal gland. Whenever this can occur, it is best to keep both items in the same half of the scale.

Kuder–Richardson 20 and Coefficient α

There are two problems in using split-half reliability to determine which items to retain. First, as we have just seen, there are many ways to divide a test; and second, it does not tell us which item(s) may be contributing to a low reliability. Both of these problems are addressed with two related techniques, *Kuder–Richardson formula 20* (KR-20; Kuder and Richardson 1937) and *Coefficient α* (also called Cronbach's alpha; Cronbach 1951).

KR-20 is appropriate for scales with items which are answered dichotomously, such as 'true—false', 'yes—no', 'present—absent', and so forth. To compute it, the proportion of people answering positively to each of the questions and the standard deviation of the total score must be known, and then put into the formula

$$\text{KR-20} = \frac{n}{n-1}\left(1 - \frac{\Sigma\, p_i q_i}{\sigma_T^2}\right),$$

where n is the number of items, p_i is the proportion answering correctly to question i, $q_i = (1 - p)$ for each item, and σ_T is the standard deviation of the total score.

Cronbach's α (alpha) is an extension of KR-20, allowing it to be used when there are more than two response alternatives. If α were used with dichotomous items, the result would be identical to that obtained with

KR-20. The formula for α is very similar to KR-20, except that the standard deviation for each item (σ_i) is substituted for $p_i q_i$:

$$\alpha = \frac{n}{n-1}\left(1 - \frac{\Sigma\,\sigma_i^2}{\sigma_T^2}\right).$$

Conceptually, both equations give the average of all of the possible split-half reliabilities of a scale. Their advantage in terms of scale development is that, especially with the use of computers, it is possible to do them n times, each time omitting one item. If KR-20 or α increases significantly when a specific item is left out, this would indicate that its exclusion would increase the homogeneity of the scale.

Discriminatory power

The issue of conflicting demands between scale homogeneity and utility crops up again within the context of the *discriminatory power* of a scale. In many situations, a scale is used to discriminate among people and spread them out as much as possible along a continuum. This is most evident in school-based tests, where the aim is to differentiate among students, all of whom may in fact be passing. The purpose of the test is to rank the students from those who are doing the best down to those whose work is only marginally acceptable or even unsatisfactory. Similarly, a rheumatologist gets much more useful information by counting the number of inflamed joints, rather than simply dichotomizing patients into two groups; inflamed and not inflamed.

To be most effective in this regard, the entire range of the scale should be used, with an equal number of people at each level; that is, the distribution of scores should be rectangular across the entire range. One index of this discriminating ability is Ferguson's δ (Ferguson 1949), defined as

$$\delta = \frac{(k+1)\,(N^2 - \Sigma f_i^2)}{kN^2},$$

where k is the number of items, N is the number of subjects, and f_i is the number of people attaining score i.

The value of δ ranges between 0, when all subjects get the same score, and +1.0, when the subjects are equally divided among all possible scores, as seen in Figure 5.1. However, in order to achieve high values for δ, the scale must include very easy items as well as very difficult ones, which tends to decrease the internal consistency of the scale. Thus, an increase in the discriminatory power of a scale may be at the expense of lowering the homogeneity of the items.

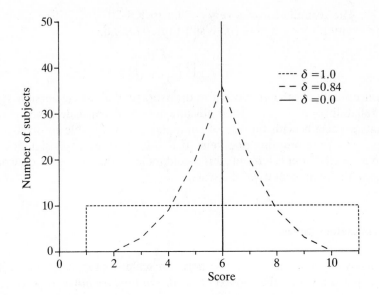

Fig. 5.1. Values of δ for different distributions of score results.

Multifactor inventories

If the scale is one part of an inventory which has a number of other scales (usually called 'multifactor' or 'multidimensional' inventories), more sophisticated item analytic techniques are possible. The first is an extension of the item—total procedure, in which the item is correlated with its scale total, *and with the totals of all of the other scales*. The item should meet the criteria outlined above for a single index; additionally, this correlation should be higher than with any of the scales it is *not* included in.

The second technique is *factor analysis*. Very briefly, this statistic is predicated on the belief that a battery of tests can be described in terms of a smaller number of underlying factors. For example, assume students were given five tests: vocabulary, word fluency, verbal analogies, mechanical reasoning, and arithmetic. It might be expected that their scores on the first three tasks would be correlated with one another, that the last two would be correlated, but that the two sets of scores would not necessarily be related to each other. That is, high scores on the first three may or may not be associated with high scores on the latter two. We would postulate that the first group reflected a 'verbal' factor, and the second a 'reasoning' one. (For more details presented in a non-mathematical fashion, see Norman and Streiner 1986; for even more detail, see Harman 1976).

In an analogous manner, each item in a multifactorial test could be treated as an individual 'test'. Ideally, then, there should be as many factors as separate scales in the inventory. The item should 'load on' (i.e., be correlated with) the scale it belongs to, and not on any other one. If it loads on the 'wrong' factor, or on two or more factors, then it is likely that it may be tapping something other than what the developer intended, and should be either rewritten or discarded.

More recent developments in factor analysis allow the test developer to specify beforehand what he or she thinks the final structure of the test should look like. The results show how closely the observed pattern corresponds to this hypothesized pattern (Darton 1980). Although factor analysis has been used quite often with dichotomous items, this practice is highly suspect, and can lead to quite anomalous results (Comrey 1978).

Putting it all together

In outline form, these are the steps involved in the initial selection of items:

A. Pre-test the items to ensure that they:
   1. are comprehensible to the target population,
   2. are unambiguous, and
   3. ask only a single question.
B. Eliminate or rewrite any items which do not meet these criteria, and pretest again.
C. Discard items endorsed by very few (or very many) subjects.
D. Check for the internal consistency of the scale using:
   1. Item–Total correlation
      (a) Correlate each item with the scale total omitting that item.
      (b) Eliminate or rewrite any with Pearson r's less than 0.20.
      (c) Rank order the remaining ones and select items starting with the highest correlation.
                                or
   2. Coefficient α or KR-20
      (a) Calculate α eliminating one item at a time.
      (b) Discard any item where α significantly increases.
E. Check that all the item response categories are endorsed with relatively the same frequency, using δ or some equivalent measure.
F. For multiscale questionnaires, check that the item is in the 'right' scale by:
   1. Correlating it with the totals of all the scales, eliminating items which correlate more highly on scales other than the one it belongs to; or

2. Factor-analysing the questionnaire, eliminating items which load more highly on other factors than the one it should belong to.

References

Allen, G. I., Breslow, L., Weissman, A., and Nisselson, H. (1954). Interviewing versus diary keeping in eliciting information in a morbidity survey. *American Journal of Public Health*, **44**, 919–27.

Allen, M. J., and Yen, W. M. (1979). *Introduction to measurement theory*. Brooks/Cole, Monterey CA.

Comrey, A. L. (1978). Common methodological problems in factor analysis. *Journal of Consulting and Clinical Psychology*, **46**, 648–59.

Cronbach, L. J. (1951). Coefficient alpha and the internal structure of tests. *Psychometrika*, **16**, 297–334.

Dale, E., and Eichholz, G. (1960). *Children's knowledge of words*. Ohio State University, Columbus OH.

Darton, R. A. (1980). Rotation in factor analysis. *The Statistician*, **29**, 167–94.

Ferguson, G. A. (1949). On the theory of test development. *Psychometrika*, **14**, 61–8.

Flesch, R. (1948). A new readability yardstick. *Journal of Applied Psychology*, **32**, 221–33.

Fry, E. A. (1968). A readability formula that saves time. *Journal of Reading*, **11**, 513–16.

Harman, H. H. (1976). *Modern factor analysis* (3rd edn). University of Chicago Press, Chicago.

Havlicek, L. L., and Peterson, N. L. (1977). Effect of the violation of assumptions upon significance levels of the Pearson *r*. *Psychological Bulletin*, **84**, 373–77.

Holden, R. R., Fekken, G. C., and Jackson, D. N. (1985). Structured personality test item characteristics and validity. *Journal of Research in Personality*, **19**, 386–94.

Jackson, D. N. (1970). A sequential system for personality scale development. In *Current topics in clinical and community psychology*, (ed. C. D. Spielberger) Vol. 2, pp. 61–96. Academic Press, New York.

Jackson, D. N. (1984). *Personality Research Form manual*. Research Psychologists Press, Port Huron MI.

Kline, P. (1986). *A handbook of test construction*. Methuen, London.

Kuder, G. F., and Richardson, M. W. (1937). The theory of estimation of test reliability. *Psychometrika*, **2**, 151–60.

McLaughlin, G. H. (1969). SMOG grading: A new readability formula. *Journal of Reading*, **12**, 639–46.

Norman, G. R., and Streiner, D. L. (1986). *PDQ statistics*. B. C. Decker, Toronto.

Nunnally, J. C., Jr. (1970). *Introduction to psychological measurement*. McGraw-Hill, New York.

Nunnally, J. C., Jr. (1978). *Psychometric theory* (2nd edn). McGraw-Hill, New York.

Payne, S. L. (1954) *The art of asking questions*. Princeton University Press, Princeton NJ.

Radloff, L. S. (1977). The CES-D scale: A self-report depression scale for research in the general population. *Applied Psychological Measurement*, **1**, 385–401.

Schriesheim, C. A., and Hill, K. D. (1981). Controlling acquiescence response bias by item reversals: The effect on questionnaire validity. *Educational and Psychological Measurement*, **41**, 1101–14.

Taylor, W. L. (1957). 'Cloze' readability scores as indices of individual differences in comprehension and aptitude. *Journal of Applied Psychology*, **41**, 19–26.

6

Biases in responding

When an item is included in a questionnaire or scale, it is usually under the assumption that the respondent will answer honestly. However, there has been considerable research, especially since the 1950s, showing that there are numerous factors which may influence a response, making it a less than totally accurate reflection of reality. The magnitude and seriousness of the problem depends very much on the nature of the instrument and the conditions under which it is used. At the extreme, questionnaires may end up over- or under-estimating the prevalence of a symptom or disease; or the validity of the scale may be seriously jeopardized.

Some scale developers bypass the entire problem of responder bias by asserting that their instruments are designed merely to differentiate between groups. In this situation, the truth or falsity of the answer is irrelevant, as long as one group responds in one direction more often than does another group. According to this position, responding 'yes' to an item such as 'I like sports magazines' would not be interpreted as accurately reflecting the person's reading preferences. The item's inclusion in the test is predicated solely on the fact that one group of people *says* it likes these magazines more often than do other groups. This purely empirical approach to scale development reached its zenith in the late 1940s and 1950s, but may still be found underlying the construction of some measures.

However, with the gradual trend toward instruments which are more grounded in theory, this approach to scale construction has become less appealing. The objective now is to reduce bias in responding as much as possible. In this chapter, we will examine some of the sources of error, what effects they may have on the scale, and how to minimize them.

The differing perspectives

The people who develop a scale, those who use it in their work, and the ones who are asked to fill it out, all approach scales from different perspectives, for different reasons, and with differing amounts of information about the instrument. For the person administering the instrument, a specific answer to a given question is often of little interest. That item may be just one of many on a scale, where the important information is the total score, and there is little regard for the individual items which have contributed to it. In other situations, the responses may be aggregated across dozens or hundreds of subjects, so that the individual person's answers are buried in a mass of those from other anonymous subjects. Further, what the questioner wants is 'truth'—did the person have this symptom or not, ever engage in this behaviour or not, and so forth. The clinician cannot help the patient, or the researcher discover important facts, unless honest answers are given. Moreover, the assessment session is perceived, at least in the assessors' minds, as non-judgmental and their attitude as disinterested. This may appear so obvious to scale developers that it never occurs to them that the responents may perceive the situation from another angle.

The respondents' perspectives, however, are often quite different. They are often unaware that the individual items are ignored in favour of the total score. Even when told that their responses will be scored by a computer, it is quite common to find marginal notes explaining or elaborating their answers. Thus, it appears that respondents treat each item as important in its own right, and often believe that their answers will be read and evaluated by another person.

Additionally, their motivation may include the very natural tendency to be seen in a good light; or to be done with this intrusion in their lives as quickly as possible; or to ensure that they receive the help they feel they need. As we will discuss, these and other factors may influence the response given.

Social desirability and faking good

A person's answer to an item like, 'During an average day, how much alcohol do you consume?' or 'I am a shy person' may not correspond to what an outside observer would say about that individual. In many cases, people give a socially desirable answer; the drinker may minimize his daily intake, or the retiring person may deny it, believing it is better to be outgoing. As *social desirability* is commonly conceptualized, the subject is not deliberately trying to deceive or lie; he or she is unaware of this tendency to put the best foot forward (Edwards 1957). When the person *is* aware and is intentionally attempting to create a false positive impression, it is called *faking good*. Although conceptually different, the two biases create similar problems for the scale developer, and have similar solutions.

Social desirability (SD) depends on many factors: the individual, the person's sex and cultural background, the specific question, and the context in which the item is asked; e.g. face-to-face interview versus an anonymous questionnaire. A debate has raged for many years whether SD is a trait (whereby the person responds in the desirable direction irrespective of the context) or a state (dependent more on the question and the setting). While the jury is still out, two suggestions have emerged: SD should be minimized whenever possible, and the person's propensity to respond in this manner should be assessed whenever it may affect how he or she answers (e.g. Anastasi 1982; Jackson 1984).

If answers are affected by social desirability, the validity of the scale may be jeopardized for two reasons. First, if the object of the questionnaire is to gather factual information, such as the prevalence of a disorder, behaviour, or feeling, then the results obtained may not reflect the true state of affairs. The prime example of this would be items tapping socially sanctioned acts, like drug taking, premarital sexual relations, or abortions; but SD may also affect responses to embarrassing, unpopular, or 'unacceptable' feelings, such as anger towards one's parents, or admitting to voting for the party which lost the last election (or won, depending on recent events). In a similar fashion, the occurrence of positive or socially desired behaviours may be overestimated.

The second problem, to which we will return in Chapter 10, involves what is called the 'discriminant validity' of a test. Very briefly, if a scale correlates highly with one factor (e.g. SD), then that limits how highly it can correlate with the factor which the scale was designed to assess. Further, the theoretical rationale of the scale is undermined, since the most parsimonious explanation of what the test is measuring would be 'social desirability', rather than anything else.

The social desirability of an item can be assessed in a number of ways. One method is to correlate each item on a new instrument with a scale specifically designed to measure this tendency. Jackson (1970) has developed an index called the *Differential Reliability Index* (DRI), defined as

$$\text{DRI} = \sqrt{(r_{is}^2 - r_{id}^2)},$$

where r_{is} is the item-scale correlation, and r_{id} is the item–SD correlation.

The DRI in essence is the difference between the item–total correlation and the item–SD correlation. Any item which is more highly 'saturated' on SD than with its scale total will result in a DRI approaching zero (note that if r_{id} is ever larger than r_{is}, DRI is undefined). Such an item should either be rewritten or discarded.

A number of scales have been developed to specifically measure the tendency to give socially desirable answers. These include the Crowne and Marlowe (1960) *Social Desirability Scale*, which is perhaps the most widely used such instrument; the *Desirability* (DY) scale on the *Personality Research Form* (Jackson 1984); and one developed by Edwards (1957). These are sometimes given in conjunction with other scales, not so much in order to develop a new instrument, as to see if SD is affecting the subject's responses. If it is not, then there is little to be concerned about; if so, though, there is little that can be done after the fact except to exercise caution in interpreting the results. Unfortunately, the correlations among the social desirability scales are low, indicating that they are tapping different things, and that the results obtained using one scale may not be comparable to those using another SD scale. This leaves the scale constructor in something of a quandary, knowing which if any SD scale to use. Most people use the Crowne and Marlowe scale, if more by habit and tradition than because of its psychometric superiority. Unless there are compelling reasons to use another index, this is probably as good a choice as any.

A second method to measure and reduce SD, used by McFarlane *et al.* (1981) in the development of their *Social Relations Scale*, is to administer the scale twice; once using the regular instructions to the subjects regarding its completion, and then asking them to fill it in as they would like things to be, or in the best of all possible worlds. This involved asking them first to list whom they talk to about issues that come up in their lives in various areas. A few weeks later (by which time they should have forgotten their original responses), they were asked to complete it 'according to what you consider to be good or ideal circumstances'. If the scores on any item did not change from the first to the second administration, it was assumed that its original answer was dictated more by SD than by the true state of affairs (or was at the 'ceiling' and could not detect any improvement). In either case, the item failed to satisfy at least one desired psychometric property, and was eliminated.

The term 'faking good' is most often applied to an intentional and deliberate approach by the person in responding to personality inventories. An analogous bias in responding to items on questionnaires is called 'prestige bias' (Oppenheim 1966). To judge from responses on questionnaires, nobody watches game shows or soap operas on TV, despite their obvious popularity; everyone watches only educational and cultural programmes. Their only breaks from these activities are to attend concerts, visit museums, and brush their teeth four or five times each day. (One can only wonder why the concert halls are empty and dentists' waiting rooms are full.)

Whyte (1956, p. 197), only half in jest, gave some advice to business people who had to take personality tests in order for them to advance up the company ladder. He wrote that, in order to select the best reply to a question, the person should repeat to himself:

- I loved my father and my mother, but my father a little bit more.
- I like things pretty well the way they are.
- I never much worry about anything.
- I don't care for books or music much.
- I love my wife and children.
- I don't let them get in the way of company work.

Since faking good and the prestige bias are more volitional than social desirability, they are easier to modify through instructions and careful wording of the items. The success of these tactics, though, is still open to question.

Deviation and faking bad

The opposite of socially desirable responding and faking good are *deviation* and *faking bad*. These latter two phenomena have been less studied than their positive counterparts, and no scales to assess them are in wide use. Deviation is a concept introduced by Berg (1967) to explain (actually, simply to name) the tendency to respond to test items with deviant responses. As is the case for faking good, faking bad occurs primarily within the context of personality assessment, although this may happen any time a person feels he or she may avoid an unpleasant situation (such as the military draft) by looking bad.

Both SD (or perhaps faking good) and deviance (or faking bad) occur together in an interesting phenomenon called the 'hello–goodbye' effect. Before an intervention, a person may present himself in as bad a light as possible, thereby hoping to qualify for the program, and impressing the staff with the seriousness of his problems. At termination, he may want to 'please' the staff with his improvement, and so may minimize any problems. The result is to make it appear that there has been improvement when none has occurred, or to magnify any effects which did occur. This effect was originally described in psychotherapy research, but it may arise whenever a subject is assessed on two occasions, with some intervention between the administrations of the scale.

Three techniques have been proposed to minimize the effects of these different biases. One method is to try to disguise the intent of the test, so the subject does not know what is actually being looked for. Rotter's scale to measure locus of control (Rotter 1966), for example, is called the *Personal Reaction Inventory*, a vague title which conveys little about the purpose of the instrument. (But then again, neither does 'locus of control'.)

However, this deception is of little use if the content of the items themselves reveals the objective of the scale. Thus, the second method consists of using 'subtle' items, ones where the respondent is unaware of the specific trait or behaviour being tapped. The item may still have face validity, since the respondent could feel that the question is fair and relevant; however, its actual relevance may be to some trait other than that assumed by the answerer (Holden and Jackson 1979). For example, the item, 'I would enjoy racing motorcycles' may appear to measure preferences for spending one's leisure time, while in fact it may be on an index of risk-taking. The difficulty with this technique, though, is that the psychometric properties of subtle items are usually poorer than those of obvious ones, and often do not measure the traits for which they were originally intended (Burkhart *et al.* 1976; Jackson 1971).

The third method of minimizing social desirability bias, especially regarding illegal, immoral, or embarrassing behaviours, is called the *random response technique* (Warner 1965). In the most widely used of many variants of the technique, the respondent is handed a card containing two items; one neutral and one sensitive. For example, the questions can be:

A. I own a VCR.

B. I have used street drugs within the past six months.

The respondent is also given a device which randomly selects an A or a B. This can be as simple as a coin, or a spinner mounted on a card divided into two zones, each labelled with one of the letters. He or she is told to flip the coin (or spin the arrow), and truthfully answer whichever item is indicated; the interviewer is not to know *which* question has been selected, only the response.

In practice, only a portion of the respondents are given these items; the remaining subjects are asked the neutral question directly in order to determine the prevalence of 'True' responses to it in the sample. When two or more such items are used, half of the group will be given the random response technique on half of the questions, and asked about the neutral stems for the remaining items; while this would be reversed for the second half of the sample. An alternative is to use a neutral item where the true prevalence is well known, such as the proportion of families owning two cars or with three children. Of course, the scale developer must be quite sure that the sample is representative of the population on which the prevalence figures were derived.

With this information, the proportion of people answering 'true' to the sensitive item (p_s) can be estimated using the equation

$$p_s = [p_t - (1 - P) p_d]/P$$

where p_t is the proportion of people who answered 'true', p_d is the proportion saying 'true' to the neutral item on direct questioning, and P is the probability of selecting the sensitive item.

The probability of selecting the sensitive item (P) is 50 per cent using a coin toss, but can be modified with other techniques. For example, the two zones on the spinner can be divided so that A covers only 30 per cent and B 70 per cent. Another modification uses two colours of balls drawn from an urn; here, the proportion of each colour (representing each stem) can be set at other than 50 per cent. The closer P is to 1.0, the smaller the sample size needed to get an accurate estimate of p_s, but the technique begins to resemble direct questioning, and anonymity becomes jeopardized.

The advantage of the random response technique is that it gives a more accurate estimate of the true prevalence of these sensitive behaviours than does direct questioning. For example, nine times as many women reported having had an abortion when asked with the random response method as compared with traditional questioning (Shimizu and Bonham 1978). However, there are some penalties associated with this procedure. First, it is most easily done in face-to-face interviews, although it is possible over the telephone. Second, since it is not known which subjects responded to each stem, the answers cannot be linked to other information from the questionnaire. Third, the calculated prevalence depends upon three estimates: the proportion of subjects responding to the sensitive item; the proportion answering 'true'; and the proportion of people who respond 'true' to the neutral stem. Since each of these is measured with error, a much larger sample size is required to get stable estimates.

Yea-saying or acquiescence

Yea-saying, also call *acquiescence bias*, is the tendency to give positive responses, such as 'true', 'like', 'often', or 'yes', to a question (Couch and Keniston 1960). At its most extreme, the person responds in this way irrespective of the content of the item, so that even mutually contradictory statements are endorsed. Thus, the person may respond 'true' to two items like 'I always take my medication on time,' and 'I often forget to take my pills.' At the opposite end of the spectrum are the 'nay-sayers.' It is believed that this tendency is more or less normally distributed, so that relatively few people are at the extremes, but that many people exhibit this trait to lesser degrees.

No specific scales have been developed to measure yea-saying or nay-saying. Rather, some people (see for example Phillips and Clancy 1970) simply count the number of items on a scale answered positively or negatively by each subject. The usual way to correct for this potential bias is to have an equal number of items keyed in the positive and negative directions. A scale for compliance with medication, then, would be randomly divided so that 'true' on half of the items would reflect compliance, as would 'false' on the remaining ones. As mentioned in Chapter 5, however, the items should be balanced with respect to how they are *keyed*, but negatively *worded* items should be avoided.

End-aversion, positive skew, and halo

In addition to the distortions already mentioned, scales which are scored on a continuum, such as visual analogue and Likert scales, are prone to other types of biases. These include end-aversion bias, positive skew, and the halo effect.

End-aversion bias

End-aversion bias, which is also called the *central tendency bias*, refers to the reluctance of some people to use the extreme categories of a scale. It is based in part on people's difficulty in making absolute judgements, since situations without mitigating or extenuating circumstances rarely occur. The problem is similar to the one some people have in responding to 'true—false' items; they often want to say, 'It all depends,' or 'Most of the time, but not always.' The effect of this bias is to reduce the range of possible responses. Thus, if the extremes of a five-point Likert scale are labelled 'always' and 'never,' an end-aversion bias would render this a three-point scale, with the resulting loss of sensitivity and reliability.

There are two ways of dealing with the end-aversion bias. The first is to avoid absolute statements at the end-points; using 'almost never' and 'almost always' instead of 'never' and 'always.' The problem with this approach is that data may be thrown away; some people may *want* to respond with absolutes, but not allowing them to dilutes their answers with less extreme ones. The advantage is a greater probability that all categories will be used.

The second, and opposite, tack is to include 'throw away' categories at the ends. If the aim is to have a seven-point scale, then nine alternatives are provided, with the understanding that the extreme boxes at the ends will rarely be checked, but are there primarily to serve as anchors. This more or less ensures that all seven categories of interest will be used, but may lead to the problem of devising more adjectives if each box is labelled.

Positive skew

It often happens, though, that the responses are not evenly distributed over the range of alternatives, but show a positive *skew* toward the favourable end. This situation is most acute when a rating scale is used to evaluate students or staff. For example, Linn (1979) found that the mean score on a five-point scale was 4.11 rather than 3.00, and the scores ranged between 3.30 and 4.56—the lower half of the scale was never used. Similarly, Cowles and Kubany (1959) asked raters to determine if a student was in the lower one-fifth, top one-fifth, or middle three-fifths of the class. Despite these explicit instructions, 31 per cent were assigned to the top fifth and only 5 per cent to the bottom one-fifth.

This may reflect the feeling that since these students survived the hurdles of admission into university and then into professional school, the 'average' student is really quite exceptional. It is then difficult to shift sets, so that 'average' is relative to the other people in the normative group, rather than the general population.

The effect of skew is to produce a *ceiling effect*; since most of the marks are clustered in only a few boxes at one extreme, the scores are very near the top of the scale. This means that it is almost impossible to detect any improvement, or to distinguish among various grades of excellence.

A few methods have been proposed to counteract this bias, all based on the fact that 'average' need not be in the middle. Since no amount of instruction or training appears to be able to shake an evaluator's belief that the average person under his or her supervision is far above average, the aim of a scale is then to differentiate among degrees of excellence. Using a traditional Likert scale, like:

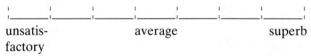

    unsatis-   average   superb
    factory

will result in most of the scores bunching in the three right-most boxes (or two, if an end-aversion is also present). However, we can shift the centre to look like this:

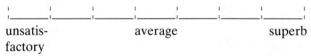

    unsatis- average   superb
    factory

This gives the evaluator five boxes above average, rather than just three.

Another strategy is to capitalize on the fact that the truly superb students or employees need little feedback, except to continue doing what they have been all along, while the unsatisfactory ones are readily apparent to all evaluators even without scales. Rather, we should use the scale to differentiate among the majority of people who fall between these extremes. In this situation, the middle is expanded, at the expense of the ends:

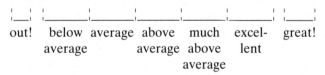

    out!   below average above   much   excel- great!
           average   average above   lent
                                   average

Note that this version clearly distinguishes the extremes, and offsets 'average'; many other variations on this theme are possible, reflecting the needs and philosophies of the program.

Halo

Halo is a phenomenon first recognized 80 years ago (Wells 1907), whereby judgements made on individual aspects of a person's performance are influenced by the rater's overall impression of the person. Thorndike (1920), who named this effect, gave what is still the best description of it: 'The judge seems intent on reporting his final opinion of the strength, weakness, merit, or demerit of the personality as a whole, rather than on giving as discriminating a rating as possible for each separate characteristic' (p. 447). For example, if a resident is well regarded by a staff physician, then the resident will be evaluated highly in all areas. Conversely, a resident who is felt to be weak in clinical skills, for example, can do no right, and will receive low scores in all categories. To some degree, this reflects reality; people who are good at one thing tend to do well in related areas. Also, many of the individual categories are dependent upon similar traits or behaviours: the ability to establish rapport with patients likely is dependent on the same skills that are involved in working with nurses and other staff. Cooper (1981) refers to this real correlation among categories as 'true halo'.

However, the ubiquity of this phenomenon and the very high intercorrelations among many different categories indicate that more is going on: what Cooper calls 'illusory halo', and what we commonly refer to when we speak of the 'halo effect'. There have been many theories proposed to explain illusory halo, but many simply boil down to the fact that raters are unable to evaluate people along more than a few dimensions. Very often, one global, summary rating scale about the person conveys as much information as do the individual scales about each aspect of the person's performance.

Many of the techniques proposed to minimize illusory halo involve factors other than the scale itself, such as the training of raters, basing the evaluations on larger samples of behaviour, and using more than one evaluator (e.g. Cooper 1981). The major aspect of scale design which may reduce this effect is the use of behaviourally-anchored ratings (BARs); instead of simply stating 'below average', for example, concrete examples are used, either as part of the descriptors themselves, or on a separate instruction page (e.g. Streiner 1985). This gives the raters concrete meaning for each level on the scale, reducing the subjective element and increasing agreement among raters.

Framing

Another bias, which particularly affects econometric scaling methods, is called *framing* (Kahneman and Tversky 1984). The name refers to the fact that the person's choice between two alternative states depends on how these states are framed. For example, consider the situation where an outbreak of influenza is expected to kill 600 people in the country. The subject must choose between two programs:

Program A: 200 people will be saved.

Program B: There is a one-third probability that 600 people will be
          saved, and two-thirds that nobody will be saved.

Nearly 75 per cent of subjects prefer Program A—assurance that 200
people will be saved—rather than the situation which offers the possibility
that everyone could be saved, but at the risk of saving no one. Now consider presenting the same situation, but offering two different programs:

Program C: 400 people will die.

Program D: There is a one-third probability that nobody will die, and
          two-thirds that 600 will die.

Programs A and C are actually the same, as are B and D; all that differs is
how the situations are presented (or 'framed'). In A, the number of survi-
vors is explicitly stated, and the number who die (400) is implicit; this is
reversed in C, where the number who die is given, but not the number who
live. From a purely arithmetic point of view, the proportion of people opt-
ing for C, then, should be similar to those who choose A. In fact, over 75 per
cent select program D rather than C, the exact reverse of the first situation.

Kahneman and Tversky explain these seemingly contradictory results by
postulating that people are 'risk averse' when gain is involved and 'risk
takers' in loss situations. That is, when offered the possibility of a gain
(saving lives, winning a bet, and so on), people tend to take the safer route
of being sure they gain something rather than the riskier alternative of perhaps getting much more, but possibly losing everything. In loss situations,
though, such as choosing between Programs C and D, people will gamble
on minimizing their losses (although there is the risk that they can lose
everything), rather than taking the certain situation that they will lose
something.

The problem that this poses for the designer of questionnaires is that the
manner in which a question is posed can affect the results that are
obtained. For example, if the researchers were interested in physicians'
attitudes toward a new operation or drug, they may get very different
answers if they said that the incidence of morbidity was 0.1 per cent, as
opposed to saying that there was a 99.9 per cent chance that nothing
untoward would occur.

In conclusion, the safest strategy for the test developer is to assume that
all of these biases are operative, and take the necessary steps to minimize
them whenever possible.

References

Anastasi, A. (1982). *Psychological testing* (5th edn). Macmillan, New York.

Berg, I. A. (1967). The deviation hypothesis: A broad statement of its assumptions
    and postulates. In *Response set in personality assessment* (ed. I. A. Berg) pp.
    146–90. Aldine, Chicago.

Burkhart, B. R., Christian, W. L., and Gynther, M. D. (1976). Item subtlety and faking on the MMPI: A paradoxical relationship. *Journal of Personality Assessment*, **42**, 76–80.

Cooper, W. H. (1981). Ubiquitous halo. *Psychological Bulletin*, **90**, 218–44.

Couch, A., and Keniston, K. (1960). Yeasayers and naysayers: Agreeing response set as a personality variable. *Journal of Abnormal and Social Psychology*, **60**, 151–74.

Cowles, J. T., and Kubany, A. J. (1959). Improving the measurement of clinical performance in medical students. *Journal of Clinical Psychology*, **15**, 139–42.

Crowne, D. P., and Marlowe, D. (1960). A new scale of social desirability independent of psychopathology. *Journal of Consulting Psychology*, **24**, 349–54.

Edwards, A. L. (1957). *The social desirability variable in personality assessment and research*. Dryden, New York.

Holden, R. R., and Jackson, D. N. (1979). Item subtlety and face validity in personality assessment. *Journal of Consulting and Clinical Psychology*, **47**, 459–68.

Jackson, D. N. (1970). A sequential system for personality scale development. In *Current topics in clinical and community psychology* (ed. C. D. Spielberger), Vol. 2 pp. 61–96. Academic Press, New York.

Jackson, D. N. (1971). The dynamics of structured personality tests: 1971. *Psychological Review*, **78**, 229–48.

Jackson, D. N. (1984). *Personality Research Form manual*. Research Psychologists Press, Port Huron MI.

Kahneman, D., and Tversky, A. (1984). Choices, values, and frames. *American Psychologist*, **39**, 341–50.

Linn, L. (1979). Interns' attitudes and values as antecedents of clinical performance. *Journal of Medical Education*, **54**, 238–40.

McFarlane, A. H., Neale, K. A., Norman, G. R., Roy, R. G., and Streiner, D. L. (1981). Methodological issues in developing a scale to measure social support. *Schizophrenia Bulletin*, **7**, 90–100.

Oppenheim, A. N. (1966). *Questionnaire design and attitude measurement*. Heinemann, London.

Phillips, D. L., and Clancy, K. J. (1970). Response biases in field studies of mental illness. *American Sociological Review*, **35**, 503–15.

Rotter, J. (1966). Generalized expectancies for internal versus external control of reinforcement. *Psychological Monographs: General and Applied*, **80** (1, Whole No. 609).

Shimizu, I. M., and Bonham, G. S. (1978). Randomized response technique in a national survey. *Journal of the American Statistical Association*, **73**, 35–9.

Streiner, D. L. (1985). Global rating scales. In *Assessing clinical competence* (eds. V. R. Neufeld and G. R. Norman), pp. 119–41. Springer, New York.

Thorndike, E. L. (1920). A constant error in psychological ratings. *Journal of Applied Psychology*, **4**, 25–9.

Warner, S. L. (1965). Randomized response: A survey technique for eliminating evasive answer bias. *Journal of the American Statistical Association*, **60**, 63–9.

Wells, F. L. (1907). A statistical study of literary merit. *Archives of Psychology*,
    1(7).
Whyte, W. H., Jr. (1956). *The organization man*. Simon and Schuster, New York.

7

From items to scales

Some scales consist of just one item, such as a visual analogue scale, on which a person may rate his or her pain on a continuum from 'no pain at all' to 'the worst imaginable pain.' However, the more usual and desirable approach is to have a number of items to assess a single underlying characteristic. This then raises the issue of how we combine the individual items into a scale, and then express the final score in the most meaningful way.

By far the easiest solution is to simply add the scores on the individual items and leave it at that. In fact, this is the approach used by many scales. The *Beck Depression Inventory* (BDI; Beck *et al.* 1961), for instance, consists of 21 items, each scored on a 0–3 scale, so the final score can range between 0 and 63. This approach is conceptually and arithmetically simple, and makes few assumptions about the individual items; the only implicit assumption is that the items are equally important in contributing to the total score.

Since this approach is so simple, there must be something wrong with it. Actually, there are two potential problems. We say 'potential' because, as will be seen later, they may not be problems in certain situations. First, some items may be more important than others, and perhaps should make a larger contribution to the total score. Second, unlike the situation in measuring blood pressure, for example, where it is expected that each of the different methods should yield exactly the same answer, no one presumes that all scales tapping activities of daily living should give the same number at the end. Under these circumstances, it is difficult, if not impossible, to compare scores on different scales, since each uses a different metric. We shall examine both of these points in some more detail.

Weighting the items

Rather than simply adding up all of the items, a scale or index may be developed which 'weights' each item differently in its contribution to the total score. There are two general approaches to doing this, theoretical and empirical. In the former, a test constructor may feel that, based on his or her understanding of the field, there are some aspects of a trait that are crucial, and others which are still interesting, but perhaps less germane. It would make at least intuitive sense for the former to be weighted more heavily than the latter. For example, in assessing the recovery of a cardiac patient, his or her ability to return to work may be seen as more important than resumption of leisure-time activities. In this case, the scale developer may multiply, or weight, the score on items relating to the first set of activities by a factor which would reflect its greater importance. (Perhaps we should mention here that the term 'weight' is preferred by statisticians to the more commonly used 'weigh'.)

The empirical approach comes from the statistical theory of multiple regression. Very briefly, in multiple regression we try to predict a score (Y) from a number of independent items (Xs), and takes the form:

$$Y = \beta_0 + \beta_1 X_1 + \beta_2 X_2 + \ldots + \beta_k X_k$$

where β_0 is a constant, and $\beta_1 \ldots \beta_k$ are the 'beta weights' for the k items.

We choose the βs to maximize the predictive accuracy of the equation. There is one optimal set, and any other set of values will result in less accuracy. In the case of a scale, Y is the trait or behaviour we are trying to predict, and the Xs are the individual items. This would indicate that a weighting scheme for each item, empirically derived, would improve the accuracy of the total score (leaving aside for the moment the question of what we mean by 'accuracy').

One obvious penalty for this greater sophistication introduced by weighting is increased computation. Each item's score must be multiplied by a constant, and these then added together; a process which is more time-consuming and prone to error than treating all items equally (i.e. giving them all weights of 1).

The question then is whether the benefits outweigh the costs. The answer is that it all depends. Wainer's (1976) conclusion was that if we eliminate items with very small β weights (that is, those that contribute little to the overall accuracy anyway), then 'it don't make no nevermind' whether the other items are weighted or not.

This was demonstrated empirically by Lei and Skinner (1980), using the Holmes and Rahe (1967) *Social Readjustment Rating Scale* (SRRS). This checklist consists of events which may have occurred in the past six months, and weighted to reflect how much adjustment would be required to adapt to it. Lei and Skinner looked at four versions of the SRRS: using the original weights assigned by Holmes and Rahe; using simply a count of the number of items endorsed, which is the same as using weights of 1 for all items; using 'perturbed' weights, where they were randomly shuffled from one item to another; and randomly assigned weights, ranging between 1 and 100.

The life events scale would appear to be an ideal situation for using weights, since there is a 100-fold difference between the lowest and highest. On the surface, at least, this differential weighting makes sense, since it seems ridiculous to assign the same weight to the death of a spouse as to receiving a parking ticket. However, they found that the correlations among these four versions was 0.97. In other words, it did not matter whether original weights, random weights, or no weights were used; people who scored high on one variant scored high on all of the others, and similarly for people who scored at the low end.

To complicate matters, though, a very different conclusion was reached by Perloff and Persons (1988). They indicated that weighting can significantly increase the predictive ability of an index, and criticize Wainer's work because he limited his discussion to situations where the β weights were evenly distributed over the interval from 0.25 to 0.75, which they feel is an improbable situation.

So, what conclusion can we draw from this argument? The answer is far from clear. It would seem that when there are at least 40 items in a scale, differential weighting contributes relatively little, except added complexity for the scorer. With fewer than 40 items (20, according to Nunnally, 1970), weighting *may* have some effect. The other consideration is that if the scale is comprised of relatively homogeneous items, where the β weights will all be within a fairly narrow range, the effect of weighting may be minimal. However, if an index consists of unrelated items, as is sometimes the case with functional status measures, then it may be worthwhile to run a multiple regression analysis and determine empirically if this improves the predictive ability of the scale.

There are two forms of weighting that are more subtle than multiplying each item by a number, and are often unintended. The first is having a different number of items for various aspects of the trait being measured, and the second is including items which are highly correlated with one another. To illustrate the first point, assume we are devising a scale to assess childhood difficulties. In this instrument, we have one item tapping into problems associated with going to bed, and five items looking at disciplinary problems. This implicitly assigns more weight to the latter category, since its potential contribution to the total score can be five times as great as the first area. Even if the parents feel that putting the child to bed is more troublesome to them than the child's lack of discipline, the scale would be weighted in the opposite direction.

There are a few ways around this problem. First, the number of items tapping each component can be equal (which assumes that all aspects contribute equally), or proportional to the importance of that area. An item-by-item matrix can be used to verify this, as was discussed in Chapter 3. A second solution is to have sub-scales, each comprised of items in one area. The total for the sub-scale would be the number of items endorsed divided by the total number of items within the sub-scale (and perhaps multiplied by 10 or 100 to eliminate decimals). The scale total is then derived by adding up these transformed sub-scale scores. In this way, each sub-scale contributes equally to the total score, even though each sub-scale may consist of a different number of items.

The second form of implicit weighting is through correlated items. Using the same example of a scale for childhood problems, assume that the section on school-related difficulties includes the following items:

1. Is often late for school
2. Talks back to the teacher
3. Often gets into fights
4. Does not obey instructions
5. Ignores the teacher

If items 2, 4, and 5 are highly correlated, then getting a score on any one of them almost automatically leads to scores on the other two. Thus, these three items are likely measuring the same thing and, as such, constitute a sub-sub-scale, and lead to problems analogous to those found with the first form of subtle weighting. The same solutions can be used, as well as a third solution: eliminating two of the items. This problem is almost universal, since we expect items tapping the same trait to be correlated; just not *too* correlated.

Unlike explicit weighting, these two forms are often unintentional. If the effects are unwanted (as they often are), special care and pre-testing the instrument are necessary to ensure that they do not occur.

Transforming the final score

The second drawback with simply adding up the items to derive a total score is that each new scale is reported on a different metric, making comparisons among scales difficult. This may not pose a problem if you are working in a brand new area, and do not foresee comparing the results to any other test. However, few such areas exist, and in most cases it is desirable to see how a person did on two different instruments. For example, the BDI, as we have said, ranges between a minimum score of 0 and a maximum of 63; while a similar test, the *Self-Rating Depression Scale* (SRDS; Zung 1965), yields a total score between 25 and 100. How can we compare a score of 23 on the former with one of 68 on the latter? It is not easy when the scores are expressed as they are.

The problem is even more evident when a test is comprised of many sub-scales, each with a different number of items. Many personality tests, like the *16PF* (Cattell et al. 1970) or the *Personality Research Form* (Jackson 1984) are constructed in such a manner, as are intelligence tests like those developed by Wechsler (1981). The resulting 'profile' of scale scores, comparing their relative elevations, would be uninterpretable if each scale were measured on a different yardstick.

The solution to this problem involves *transforming* the raw score in some way in order to facilitate interpretation. In this section, we discuss three different methods: percentiles, standard and standardized scores, and normalized scores.

Percentiles

A *percentile* is the percentage of people who score below a certain value; the lowest score is at the 0th percentile, since nobody has a lower one, while the top score is at the 99th percentile. Nobody can be at the 100th percentile, since that implies that everyone, including that person, has a lower score, an obvious impossibility. In medicine, perhaps the most widely used example of scales expressed in percentiles are developmental height and weight charts. After a child has been measured, his height is plotted on a table for children the same age. If he is at the 50th percentile, that means that he is exactly average for his age; half of all children are taller and half are shorter.

To show how these are calculated, assume a new test has been given to a large, representative sample, which is called a 'normative' or 'reference' group. If the test is destined to be used commercially, 'large' often means 1000 or more carefully selected people; for more modest aims, 'large' can mean about 100 or so. The group should be chosen so that their scores span the range you would expect to find when you finally use the test. The next step is to put the scores in *rank order*, ranging from the highest to the lowest. For illustrative purposes, suppose the normative group consists of (a ridiculously small number) 20 people. The results would look something like Table 7.1.

Starting with the highest score, a 37 for Subject 5, 19 of the 20 scores are lower, so a raw score of 37 corresponds to the 95th percentile. Subject 3 has a raw score of 21; since 12 of the 20 scores are lower, he is at the 60th percentile (i.e. 12/20). A slight problem arises when there are ties, as with Subjects 17 and 8, or 19 and 14. If there are an odd number of ties, as exists for a score of 16, we take the middle person (Subject 20 in this case), and count the number of people below. Since there are six of them, a raw score of 16 is at the 30th percentile, and all three people then get this value. If there are an even number of ties, then you will be dealing with 'halves' of a person. Thus, 8.5 people have scores lower than 17, so it corresponds to the 42.5th percentile. We continue doing this for all scores, and then rewrite the table, putting in the percentiles corresponding to each score, as in Table 7.2.

The major advantage of percentiles is that most people, even those without

Table 7.1 *Raw scores for 20 subjects on a hypothetical test*

Subject	Score	Subject	Score
5	37	19	17
13	32	14	17
2	31	1	16
15	29	20	16
17	26	7	16
8	23	6	15
10	23	11	13
3	21	16	12
12	20	4	10
18	19	9	8

Table 7.2 *The raw scores converted to percentiles*

Subject	Score	Percentile	Subject	Score	Percentile
5	37	95	19	17	42.5
13	32	90	14	17	42.5
2	31	85	1	16	35
15	29	80	20	16	35
17	26	75	7	16	35
8	23	67.5	6	15	25
10	23	67.5	11	13	20
3	21	60	16	12	10
12	20	55	4	10	5
18	18	50	9	8	0

any training in statistics or scale development, can readily understand them. However, there are a number of difficulties with this approach. One problem is readily apparent in Table 7.2; unless you have many scores, there can be fairly large jumps between the percentile values of adjacent scores. Also, it is possible that in a new sample, some people may have scores higher or lower than those in the normative group, especially if it was small and not carefully chosen. This makes interpretation of these more extreme scores problematic at best. Third, since percentiles are ordinal data, they should not be analysed using parametric statistics; means and standard deviations derived from percentiles are not legitimate.

A fourth difficulty with percentiles is a bit more subtle, but just as insidious. The distribution of percentile scores is rectangular. However, the distribution of raw test scores usually resembles a normal, or bell-shaped, curve, with most of the values clustered around the mean, and progressively fewer ones as we move out to the extremes. As a result, small differences in the middle range become exaggerated, and large differences in the tails are truncated. For example, a score of 16 corresponds to the 35th percentile, while a score just two points higher is at the 50th percentile. By contrast, a five-point difference, from 32 to 37, results in just a five-point spread in the percentiles.

Standard and standardized scores

To get around these problems with percentiles, a more common approach is to use *standard scores*. The formula to transform raw scores to standard scores is

$$z = \frac{X - \bar{X}}{\text{SD}}$$

where X is the total score for an individual, $\bar{X}$ is the mean score of the sample, and SD is the sample's standard deviation.

This 'transforms' the scale to have a mean of 0 and a standard deviation of 1, so the individual scores are expressed in standard deviation units. Moreover, since the transformation is linear, the distribution of the raw scores (ideally normal) is preserved. For example, the mean of the 20 scores in the table is 20.0, and the standard deviation is 7.75. We can convert Subject 5's score of 37 into a z-score by putting these numbers into the formula. When we do this, we find

$$z = \frac{37 - 20}{7.75} = 2.19.$$

That is, his score of 37 is slightly more than two standard deviations above the mean on this scale. Similarly, a raw score of 12 yields a z-score of -1.55, showing that this person's score is about one and a half standard deviations below the group mean.

If all test scores were expressed in this way, then we could compare results across them quite easily. Indeed, we can use this technique on raw scores from different tests, as long as we have the means and standard deviations of the tests. Then, if we received scores on two tests given to a patient at two different times, and purportedly measuring the same thing, we can see if there has been any change by transforming both of them to z-scores. As an example, we can now answer the question, how does a score of 23 on the BDI compare with 68 on the SRDS? The mean and SD of the Beck are 11.3 and 7.7, and they are 52.1 and 10.5 for the Zung. Putting the raw scores into the equation with their respective means and SDs, we find that 23 on the Beck corresponds to a z-score of 1.52, and 65 on the Zung yields a z-score of 1.51. So, although the raw scores are very different, they probably reflect similar degrees of depression.

In real life, though, we are not used to seeing scores ranging from about -3.0 to $+3.0$; we are more accustomed to positive numbers only, and whole ones at that. Very often, then, we take a second step and transform the z-score into what is called a *standardized* or *T-score*, by using the formula:

$$T = (\bar{X}' + \text{SD}')z$$

where $\bar{X}'$ is the new mean that we want the test to have, SD$'$ is the desired standard deviation, and z is the original z-score.

We can also go directly from the raw scores to the T-scores by combining this equation with that for the z-score transformation, in which case we get

$$T = \bar{X}' + \frac{(\text{SD}')\,(X - \bar{X})}{\text{SD}}.$$

A standardized or T-score is simply a z-score with a new mean and standard deviation, chosen relatively arbitrarily, and depending on custom, tradition, or just whim. For example, many personality tests use a mean of 50 and a standard deviation of 10 by convention; while the national tests for admission to university, graduate school, or professional programs use a mean of 500 and an SD of 100. Intelligence tests, for the most part, have a mean of 100 and an SD of 15. If we were developing a new IQ test, we would give it to a large normative sample and then transform each possible total raw score into a z-score. Then, setting $\bar{X}'$ to be 100 and SD$'$ to be 15, we would translate each z-score into its equivalent T-score. The result would be a new test, whose scores are directly comparable to those from older IQ tests.

The z- and T-scores do more than simply compare the results on two different tests. Like percentiles, they allow us to see where a person stands in relation to everybody else. If we assume that the scores on the test are fairly normally distributed, then we use the normal curve to determine what proportion of people score higher and lower. As a brief review, a normal curve looks like Figure 7.1. Most of the scores are clustered around the mean of the test, with progressively fewer scores as we move out to the tails. By definition, 50 per cent of the scores fall below the mean, and 50 per cent above; while 68 per cent are between -1 and $+1$ SD. That means that 84 per cent of scores fall below 1 SD—the 50 per cent below the mean plus 34 per cent between the mean and $+1$ SD. To use a concrete example, the MCAT has a mean of 500 and a standard deviation of 100. So, 68 per cent of the people have scores between 400 and 600, and 84 per cent have scores lower than 600 (meaning that 16 per cent have higher scores). We

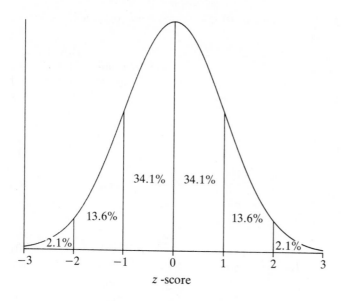

34.1% 34.1%

13.6% 13.6%

2.1% 2.1%

−3 −2 −1 0 1 2 3

z -score

Fig. 7.1. The normal curve.

can look up other values in a table of the normal distribution, which can be found in most statistics books. This is an extremely useful property of *z*- and *T*-scores, which is why many widely-used tests report their final scores in this way. Another advantage of these scores is that, since they are based on the normal curve, they often more closely meet the assumptions of parametric statistics than do either raw scores or percentiles, although it is not safe to automatically assume that standardized scores *are* normally distributed.

Any clinician who has undergone the painful process of having to re-learn normal values of laboratory tests using the SI system must wonder why standard scores are not used in the laboratory. Indeed, the problem is twofold: switching from one measurement system to another; and different values of 'normal' within each system. For example, the normal range for fasting plasma glucose used to be between 70 and 110 mg per cent, and was 1.1–4.1 ng ml^{-1} h^{-1} for plasma renin. In SI units, these same values are 3.9–6.1 mmol l^{-1} for glucose, and 0.30–1.14 ng l^{-1} s^{-1} for renin. Think how much easier life would be if the results of all these diverse tests could be expressed in a common way, such as standard or standardized scores.

Normalized scores

In order to ensure that standard and standardized scores are normally distributed, we can use other transformations which normalize the raw scores.

Table 7.3 *Percentiles transformed into normalized standard and standardized scores*

Subject	Score	Percentile	Normalized standard score (z)	Normalized standardized score (T)
5	37	95	1.65	116.5
13	32	90	1.29	112.9
2	31	85	1.04	110.4
15	29	80	0.84	108.4
17	26	75	0.67	106.7
8	23	67.5	0.45	104.5
10	23	67.5	0.45	104.5
3	21	60	0.25	102.5
12	20	55	0.13	101.3
18	18	50	0.00	100.0
19	17	42.5	−0.19	98.1
14	17	42.5	−0.19	98.1
1	16	35	−0.39	96.1
20	16	35	−0.39	96.1
7	16	35	−0.39	96.1
6	15	25	−0.67	93.3
11	13	20	−0.84	91.6
16	12	10	−1.29	87.1
4	10	5	−1.65	83.5
9	8	0	−3.00	70.0

One of the most widely used ones is the *normalized standard score*. Returning to Table 7.2, we take one further step, transforming the percentiles into standard scores from a table of the normal curve. For example, the 95th percentile corresponds to a normalized standard score of 1.65; the 90th percentile to a score of 1.29, and so on. As with non-normalized standard scores, we can, if we wish, convert these to *standardized*, normalized scores, with any desired mean and standard deviation. In Table 7.3, we have added two more columns; the first showing the transformation from percentiles to normalized standard (z) scores, and then to normalized standardized (T) scores, using a mean of 100 and a standard deviation of 10.

Age and sex norms

Some attributes, especially those assessed in adults like Peak Flow or FEV1 in respirology, show relatively little change with age and do not differ between males and females. Other factors, such as measures of lung capacity like FVC, show considerable variation with age or gender. It is well known, for example, that females are more prone to admit to depressive symptomatology than are men. The psychometric solution to this problem is relatively easy: separate norms can be developed for each sex, as was done for the Depression scale and some others on the MMPI. However, this may mask a more important and fundamental difficulty; do the sexes differ only in terms of their willingness to endorse depressive items, or does this reflect more actual depression in women? Separate norms assume that the distribution of depression is equivalent for males and females, and it is only the reporting that is different.

The opposite approach was taken by Wechsler (1958) in constructing his intelligence tests. He began with the explicit assumption that males and females do not differ on any of the dimensions that his instruments tap. During the process of developing the tests, he therefore discarded any tasks, such as spatial relations, which did show a systematic bias between the sexes.

These decisions were *theoretically founded* ones, not psychometric ones, based on the developer's conception of how these attributes exist in reality. Deciding whether sex norms should be used (as with the MMPI) or whether more endorsed items means more underlying depression (as in the Beck or Zung scales), or if the sexes *should* differ on some trait such as intelligence reflects a theoretical model. Since these are crucial in interpreting the results, they should be spelled out explicitly in any manual or paper about the instrument.

Age norms are less contentious, as developmental changes are more objective and verifiable. Some of the many examples of age-related differences are height, weight, or vocabulary. When these exist, separate norms are developed for each age group, and often age-sex group, as boys and girls develop at different rates. The major question facing the test constructor is how large the age span should be in each normative group. The answer depends to a large degree on the speed of maturation of the trait; a child should not change in his or her percentile level too much in crossing from the upper limit of one age group to the beginning of the next. If this does occur, then it is probable that the age span is too great.

Summary

We have covered three points in this chapter. First, differential weighting of items rarely is worth the trouble. Second, if a test is being developed for local use only, it would probably suffice to use simply the sum of the items. However, for more general use, and to be able to compare the results with other instruments, it is better to transform the scores into percentiles, and best to transform them into z-scores or T-scores. Third, for attributes which differ between males and females, or which show development changes, separate age or age-sex norms can be developed.

References

Beck, A. T., Ward, C. H., Mendelson, M., Mock, J., and Erbaugh, J. (1961). An inventory for measuring depression. *Archives of General Psychiatry*, **4**, 561–71.

Cattell, R. B., Eber, H. W., and Tatsuoka, M. M. (1970). *Handbook for the Sixteen Personality Factor Questionnaire (16PF)*. Institute for Personality and Ability Testing, Champaign IL.

Holmes, T. H., and Rahe, R. H. (1967). The social readjustment rating scale. *Journal of Psychosomatic Research*, **11**, 213–18.

Jackson, D. N. (1984). *Personality Research Form manual*. Research Psychologists Press, Port Huron MI.

Lei, H., and Skinner, H. A. (1980). A psychometric study of life events and social readjustment. *Journal of Psychosomatic Research*, **24**, 57–65.

Nunnally, J. C., Jr. (1970). *Introduction to psychological measurement*. McGraw-Hill, New York.

Perloff, J. M., and Persons, J. B. (1988). Biases resulting from the use of indexes: An application to attributional style and depression. *Psychological Bulletin*, **103**, 95–104.

Wainer, H. (1976). Estimating coefficients in linear models: It don't make no nevermind. *Psychological Bulletin*, **83**, 213–17.

Wechsler, D. (1958). *The measurement and appraisal of adult human intelligence* (4th edn.). Williams and Wilkins, Baltimore.

Wechsler, D. (1981). *WAIS-R manual: Wechsler Adult Intelligence Scale - Revised*. Psychological Corporation, New York.

Zung, W. K. (1965). A self-rating depression scale. *Archives of General Psychiatry*, **12**, 63–70

8

Reliability

Having completed the steps involved in creating an instrument, the investigator must now embark on empirical demonstration that the scale is measuring what was intended. A first step in this process is the assessment of *reliability*, which amounts to determining that the instrument is measuring something in a reproducible and consistent fashion.

Understanding the concept of reliability

Although the techniques for assessing reliability can become quite complex, the concept is analogous in many ways to some common practices in clinical and laboratory medicine. In the calibration of laboratory instruments, clinical laboratories routinely make an assessment of *precision*, or reproducibility of laboratory measurements, by introducing split samples and determining the variability of individual measurements. This variability is expressed as a standard deviation (SD) of the individual values around the calculated mean, so that the precision of a laboratory determination of a serum sodium may be quoted as $\pm$ 2.3 mmol l^{-1}. Because the normal range of serum sodium is of the order of 130–150 mmol l^{-1}, it is easy to judge the acceptability of this amount of laboratory error.

In clinical medicine, it is more common to examine observer *agreement* regarding the presence or absence of a particular sign or symptom, or a particular feature on a slide or radiograph. For example, we might present a series of chest films to two radiologists, and ask them to judge the presence or absence of signs of pneumoconiosis. The data might be presented as in Table 8.1 below.

In this example, the agreement between the observers is represented by the top left and bottom right cells, and equals (14 + 81)/110 or 86 per cent. This expression of reproducibility as a percentage agreement is an alternative to citing the error of measurement when the observation is categorical. As we shall see later, the use of simple agreement measures in this situation has some problems and alternatives will be suggested. Still, it is evident that this 2 × 2 table is one way of representing the concept of reproducibility.

Extending the concept a bit further, we might examine a situation where

Table 8.1   *Signs of pneumoconiosis chest X-rays*

		Observer 2		
		Present	Absent	TOTAL
Observer 1	Present	14	7	21
	Absent	8	81	89
	TOTAL	22	88	110

Table 8.2   *Stages of breast cancer*

		Observer 2				
		I	II	III	IV	TOTAL
	I	25	7	2	1	35
Observer 1	II	4	14	5	0	23
	III	3	6	17	3	29
	IV	0	1	2	10	13
	TOTAL	32	28	26	14	100

the judgement is not simply one of presence or absence, but instead is an assessment of degree. A common area is the judgement of severity of illness. In the diagnosis of cancer, the stage of the illness has a strong relationship with prognosis, and as a result, criteria have been defined for staging of many forms of cancer. Since some subjective judgement is required, it is likely that differences among observers may exist. Suppose two observers were to independently examine a series of 100 women with breast cancer, and assign a stage from I to IV, according to predefined criteria. The data might be presented as a 4 × 4 table as Table 8.2.

If we were to proceed as before, the agreement between the two observers is $(25+14+17+10)/100 = 66$ per cent, which is not very impressive. However, it is evident that, although there are 34 cases of disagreement, most of these are only one unit apart, and there is only one case where the two observers disagree by three levels. Evidently, any measure of simple agreement does not do justice to the situation, and we must devise methods to capture partial, as well as complete agreement.

Circumstances are further complicated in measurement situations where there is an assumption that the scale assesses an underlying continuum. For example, most of the rating scales we spoke of in Chapter 4 were based on five- or seven-point scales, but with an assumption that the property varied continuously, and the number of levels was, to some degree, arbitrary. If we demand perfect agreement as a measure of reproducibility, it is evident that the more categories we use, the lower the chance of achieving agreement. As a result, any measure of complete agreement would be at the mercy of the number of levels chosen.

Suppose, for example, that two observers assess a total of ten patients for some attribute (e.g., sadness) on a nine-point scale. The scores are shown in Table 8.3.

We can see that there is some variability in the scores. Scores assigned by the two observers to individual patients differ by as much as 2 units on the scale. Further, the difference between the mean scores of the observers (5.0 vs 6.0) suggests that there may be some systematic difference between them.

One approach to assessing reliability might be to examine the agreement between the two observers as we did before. In this example, agreement between observers occurred only once, with Patient 3, so we could express reliability as the proportion of cases where agreement occurred, i.e. 1/10 or 10 per cent. Such an estimate makes the situation look very bad indeed, and is not really a fair representation of the data, since an inspection of the scores seems to indicate that, although total agreement is rare, close agreement is quite common. At this point, we might distinguish between two terms which are often confused in the literature. As we have seen, the *agreement* between the two observers, where each assigns exactly the same score as the other, is quite low. Nevertheless, the *association* between the observers, where a high score by one is paralleled by a high score from the other, and a low score by one with a low score by the other, is quite high. In particular, the observers agree within one category 6 times, and within

Table 8.3 *Degree of sadness in 10 patients rated by 2 observers*

Patient	Observer 1	Observer 2	Mean
1	4	6	5.0
2	6	7	6.5
3	2	2	2.0
4	3	4	3.5
5	5	4	4.5
6	8	9	8.5
7	5	7	6.0
8	6	7	6.5
9	4	6	5.0
10	7	8	7.5
Mean	5.0	6.0	5.5

two categories 3 times, so that agreement within two categories on a seven-point scale is 100 per cent. Of course, we could continue to manipulate the categories, for example by lumping scores into broader categories like 'less than 2', '3–5', '6 or more', and create agreement figures between 10 and 100 per cent almost at will. Ironically, by creating larger categories, we will have the effect of reducing the precision of measurement, since each category is larger, but increasing the apparent agreement.

It is evident that to continue to approach the problem by examining the frequency of judgement in individual categories becomes increasingly untenable as the measure approaches an underlying continuum. Instead, we might take a second look at the laboratory approach, and see if the methods might be applied here. We would then indicate the reproducibility of the scores by determining the amount of error in an individual assessment, for example by determining the average difference between individual values and the mean value for each patient. This is analogous to the usual approach to determining instrument error in the laboratory.

This approach is also consistent with everyday experience. The knowledge that a thermometer is accurate to ±1°C provides considerable information and we could easily agree that such an instrument would be perfectly appropriate for weather forecasting, and nearly useless for monitoring body temperature. However, the reason that the measurement error alone provides useful information in the everyday world is that we share a common perception of the expected differences we will encounter in a particular situation. We know that winter temperatures in the Northern hemisphere are around 0°C and summer temperatures around 30°C (in North America) or 20°C (in Europe), so that an error of 1° is relatively small by comparison. Similarly, since the difference between a normal temperature and a moderate fever is only about 3°, the same instrument is unlikely to be useful in the clinic.

In the situation which we originally introduced, the measurement of sadness, such consensual information was conspicuously absent. We did not know the degree of difference among patients we could expect on the scale, therefore the error of measurement was of little use in making decisions regarding the adequacy of the instrument. One way to include the information about expected variability between patients would be to cite the ratio of measurement error to total variability between patients Since the total variability between patients includes both measurement error and any systematic variation between patients, this would result in a number between 0 and 1 with 0 representing a 'perfect' instrument. Such a ratio would then indicate the ability of the instrument to differentiate among patients. In practice, the ratio is turned around, and researchers calculate the ratio of variance between patients to total variance (the sum of between-patient variance and error variance), so that a 0 indicates no

reproducibility, and a 1 indicates no measurement error and perfect reproducibility. When expressed in this manner, the property is called *reliability*,
and the number between 0 and 1 the *reliability coefficient*.

Note that it is not uncommon for reliability studies to examine the mean
score of different observers, and if the means are not significantly different,
to conclude that the scale is reliable. This approach is illogical and incorrect, since any number of situations, in which there is no agreement among
observers, could result in no average difference among observer means.
For example, if the scores of observers were perfectly *inversely* correlated,
so that a '1' by the first observer was paired with a '9' by the second, and a
'9' by the first with a '1' by the second, the means of the two observers
would not differ. If the two observers assigned scores at random using the
toss of a die, again, no difference between observer means would result.
Thus, any assessment of reliability must focus on the association between
scores assigned to individual patients by different observers.

Determining the reliability of a test

In order to determine the variance due to patients, observers, and random
error, we use a technique called analysis of variance (ANOVA). The name
arises from the fact that the method takes all the variability among the 20
scores in Table 8.3 (variance) and apportions it to different sources. In this
example, there are three different sources—differences from one patient to
another, differences between the two observers, and what remains—i.e.
random error.

The variability due to *patients* is calculated by determining how much the
mean score for each patient differs from the grand mean; the mean of all
scores, which is 5.5. Theses differences are then squared and added
together. Last, since each subject's mean is based on two scores, the sum is
multiplied by two. Putting it all together we get:

$$\text{Sum of squares}_{pat} = 2[(5.0-5.5)^2 + (6.5-5.5)^2 + (2.0-5.5)^2$$
$$+ \ldots + (7.5-5.5)^2] = 66.0.$$

Similarly, we can calculate how much variance is due to the observers,
by subtracting the grand mean from the mean of each observer, and squar-
ing. Again, since each observer's mean is based on ten observations, we
multiply the sum by 10 in this case:

$$\text{Sum of squares}_{obs} = 10[(5.0-5.5)^2 + (6.0-5.5)^2] = 5.0.$$

The calculation of the random error, which is called the *error* term in
ANOVA, is a bit more complicated, and involves seeing how much each
individual score deviates from its expected value. We can use the Patient 1

—Observer 1 score as an example. First, the overall estimate of any person's score is the grand mean, 5.5. But Patient 1's mean of 5.0 is a half a point below the grand mean, so a better estimate would be $(5.5 - 0.5) = 5.0$. Last, Observer 1's mean is half a point below the grand mean as well, so the best estimate of this score would be $(5.0 - 0.5) = 4.5$. The actual score is 4.0, so the difference is assumed to be due to random error. The first term in the sum of squares would be $(4.0 - 4.5)^2$, and we can proceed similarly for the remaining 19 scores, yielding a sum of squares like:

$$\text{Sum of squares}_{err} = [(6.0{-}6.0)^2 + (5.0{-}5.5)^2 + (4.0{-}4.5)^2$$
$$+ \ldots + (8.0{-}8.0)^2] = 4.0.$$

The actual calculation uses simplifying formulae, and is carried out by computer, but it is important to understand what is being done conceptually. An ANOVA table can then be developed from the sums of squares as below in Table 8.4.

The next step is to break down the total variance in the scores into components of variance due to patients, observers, and error. It would seem that each mean square is a variance, and no further work is required, but such is not the case. Both the calculated mean square due to patients and those due to observers contain some contribution due to error variance. The easiest way to understand this concept is to imagine a situation where all patients had all the same degree of sadness, as determined by some absolute standard. Would the patients all then obtain the same scores on our sadness scale? Not at all. There would be variability in the obtained scores directly related to the amount random error present in the measurements. The relevant equations relating the mean squares (MS) to variances are below:

$$MS_{pat} = \sigma^2_{err} + 2\sigma^2_{pat}$$
$$MS_{obs} = \sigma^2_{err} + 10\sigma^2_{obs}$$
$$MS_{err} = \sigma^2_{err}.$$

From these, we can show that:

$$\sigma^2_{err} = MS_{err} = 0.44$$
$$\sigma^2_{pat} = (MS_{pat} - MS_{err})/2 = 3.44$$
$$\sigma^2_{obs} = (MS_{obs} - MS_{err})/10 = 0.45.$$

Finally, we are in a position to determine the reliability coefficient as the ratio of variance between patients to (error variance and variance between patients).

$$R = \frac{\sigma^2_{pat}}{\sigma^2_{pat} + \sigma^2_{err}} = 3.44/(3.44 + 0.44) = 0.88.$$

Table 8.4   *Analysis of variance summary table*

Source	Sum of squares	Degrees of freedom	Mean square	F
Patients	66.0	9	7.33	16.65
Observers	5.0	1	5.0	11.36
Error	4.0	9	0.44	
Total	75.0	19		

This is the classical definition of reliability. Note, however, that variance due to the observer, which amounts to a systematic difference or bias between the two observers, has been omitted. Whether this term should or should not be included is a decision which is dependent on the ultimate use of the instrument. For example, if the eventual application will always use the same two observers who were involved in the reliability study, then the two observers have been calibrated. Any score obtained from the first observer will have 0.5 added, and one from the second observer will have 0.5 subtracted. If such a correction factor is applied, then there is no reason to include this observer bias term in the reliability coefficient.

Conversely, if the two observers in the reliability study are intended as a random sample of a number of possible observers, or if no correction can be applied, then observer bias can result in a further error introduced into any individual score, and the bias term should be included in the reliability coefficient. The resulting coefficient is then

$$R = \frac{\sigma^2_{pat}}{\sigma^2_{pat} + \sigma^2_{obs} + \sigma^2_{err}} = 3.44/(3.44 + 0.45 + 0.44) = 0.794.$$

We now consider a final variation on this theme. One possible way of improving reliability (although it is already very high in this example) would be to take multiple observations and average the scores. The result of this strategy is to divide the error variance by the number of observations. So if three observers were involved and their scores averaged, the reliability of this average score is:

$$R = \frac{\sigma^2_{pat}}{\sigma^2_{pat} + (\sigma^2_{obs} + \sigma^2_{err})/3} = 3.44/[3.44 + (0.44 + 0.45)/3] = 0.921.$$

Different approaches to assessing reliability

Up to this point, we have concerned ourselves with reliability as a measure of association, examining the effect of different observers on scores. The example we have worked through included only one source of error, that which resulted from different observers' perceptions of the same behaviour. Upon reflection, we can see that there may be other sources of error or contamination in an observation of an individual patient's 'sadness'. For example, each observer may apply slightly different standards from day to day. This could be tested experimentally by videotaping a group of patients and having the observer do two ratings of the tapes a week or two apart. The resulting reliability is called an *intra-observer reliability* coefficient, since it measures variation which occurs within an observer as a result of multiple exposures to the same stimulus, as opposed to the *inter-observer* reliability we have already calculated.

Note that although many investigators maintain that the demonstration of both inter- and intra-observer reliability is a minimum requirement, this may be unnecessary. If we recognize that inter-observer reliability contains all the sources of error contributing to intra-observer reliability, in addition to any differences which may arise between observers, then it is evident that a demonstration of high inter-observer reliability is sufficient; the intra-observer reliability is bound to be higher. However, if the inter-observer reliability is low, we cannot be sure whether this arises from differences within or between observers, and it may then be necessary to continue to an intra-observer reliability study.

Often there are no observers involved in the measurement, for example, in the many self-rated tests of psychological function, pain, or disease severity. Although there are no observers, we may still be concerned about the reliability of the scale. The usual approach is to administer the scale on two occasions separated by a time interval sufficiently short that we can assume the underlying process is unlikely to have changed. This approach is called *test–retest reliability*. Of course the trick is to select an appropriate time interval: too long, and things may have changed, too short, and patients may remember their first response. Expert opinions regarding the appropriate interval vary from an hour to a year, depending on the task, but generally speaking, a retest interval of 2 to 14 days is usual.

Frequently, measures of internal consistency, as described in Chapter 5, are reported as the reliability of a test. However, since they are based on performance observed in a single sitting, there are many sources of variance which occur from day to day or between observers, which do not enter in the calculation. Because they can be calculated from routine administration of a measure, without the special requirements for two or more administrations, they appear very commonly in the literature but should be interpreted with great caution.

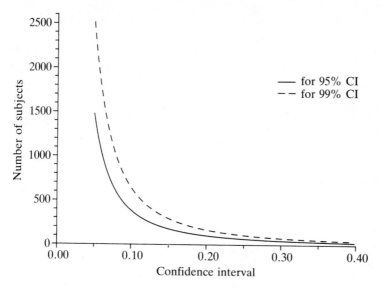

Fig. 8.1. Sample sizes for reliability studies.

Sample sizes for reliability studies

In conducting a reliability study, we are attempting to estimate the reliability coefficient with as much accuracy as possible; that, we want to be certain that the true reliability coefficient is reasonably close to the estimate we have determined. This is one form of the *confidence interval* (for further discussion consult one of the recommended statistics books). As we might expect, the larger the sample we use in the study, the smaller will be the confidence interval. The relation between sample size (*N*) and confidence interval (CI) is:

$$N = (z_{\alpha/2}/\text{CI})^2 + 3$$

where $z_{\alpha/2} = 1.96$ for a 95 per cent confidence interval and 2.54 for a 99 per cent confidence interval.

This relation is shown in the graph of Figure 8.1. From the graph, we see that to estimate a reliability coefficient with a 95 per cent CI of width 0.1, i.e. one which might extend from 0.75 to 0.85 around an estimate of 0.7 would require 387 subjects. Nunnally (1978) recommends at least 300 subjects, while Guilford (1956) and Kline (1986) are a little less demanding and recommend 200. This sample size would result in a 95 per cent CI of ±0.15.

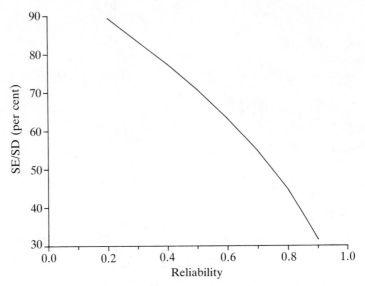

Fig. 8.2. Relation between reliability and standard error of measurement.

Interpreting the reliability coefficient

Reliability and the standard error of measurement

One difficulty with expressing the reliability coefficient as a dimensionless ratio of variances instead of an error of measurement is that it is difficult to interpret a reliability of 0.7 in terms of an individual score. However, since the reliability coefficient involves two quantities—the error variance and the variance between subjects—it is straightforward to work backwards and express the error of measurement in terms of the other two quantities. The *standard error of measurement (SEM)* is defined in terms of the standard deviation (σ) and the reliability (R) as:

$$\text{SEM} = \sigma \sqrt{(1-R)}.$$

This relationship is plotted for some values of reliability in Figure 8.2. The interpretation of this graph is that if we begin with a sample of known standard deviation and, for example, a reliability of 0.8, the error of measurement associated with any individual score is 45 per cent of the standard deviation. With a reliability of 0.5, the standard error is 70 per cent of a standard deviation, so we have improved the precision of measurement by only 30 per cent over the information we would have prior to doing any assessment of the individual at all.

Another way to interpret this is to imagine that we had a scale with a standard deviation of 10 and a reliability of 0.8. If someone's true score were 15 on the measure, then we would expect that 68 per cent of the time her observed score would fall between 15 − (10 × 0.45) and 15 + (10 × 0.45), i.e. between 10.5 and 19.57.

Standards for the magnitude of the reliability coefficient

From the previous section, it should be evident that reliability cannot be conceived of as a property which a particular instrument does or does not possess; rather any measure will have a certain degree of reliability when applied to certain populations under certain conditions. The issue which must be addressed is how much reliability is 'good enough'. Authors of textbooks on psychometric theory often make brief recommendations, usually without justification or reference to other recommendations. In fact, there can be no sound basis for such a recommendation, any more than there can be a sound basis for the decision that a certain percentage of candidates sitting an examination will fail.

For what it is worth, here are two authors' opinions for acceptable reliability for tests used to make decisions about individuals: Kelly (1927) recommended a minimum of 0.94, while Weiner and Stewart (1984) suggested 0.85.

Fortunately, some authors avoid any such arbitrary judgement. However, the majority of textbooks then make a further distinction: namely, that a test used for individual judgement should be more reliable than one used for group decisions or research purposes. There are two possible justifications for this distinction. First, the research will draw conclusions from a mean score averaged across many individuals, and the sample size will serve to reduce the error of measurement in comparison to group differences. Second, rarely will decisions about research findings be made on the basis of a single study; conclusions are usually drawn from a series of replicated studies. But a recommendation of reliability, such as attempted by Weiner and Stewart (1984), remains tenuous since a sample of 1000 can tolerate a much less reliable instrument than a sample of 10, so that the acceptable reliability is dependent on the sample size used in the research.

Reliability and the probability of misclassification

An additional problem of interpretation arising from the reliability coefficient is that it does not, of itself, indicate just how many wrong decisions (false positives or false negatives) will result from a measure with a particular reliability. There is no straightforward answer to this problem, since the probability of misclassification, when the underlying measure is continuous, relates both to the property of the instrument and to the decision of the location of the cutpoint. For example, if we had people trained to assess haemoglobin using an office haemoglobinometer and classify patients as normal or anaemic on the basis of a single random blood sample, the number of false positives and false negatives will be dependent on the reliability of the reading of a single sample, but will also depend on two other variables: where we decide to set the boundary between normal and anaemic and the base rate of anaemia in the population under study.

Some indication of the relationship between reliability and the probability of misclassification was given by Thorndike and Hagen (1969), who avoided the 'cutpoint' problem by examining the ranking of individuals. Imagine one hundred individuals who have been tested and ranked. Consider one individual ranked 25th from the top, and another ranked 50th. If the reliability is 0, there is a 50 per cent chance that the two will reverse order on repeated testing since the measure conveys no information and the ordering, as a result, is arbitrary. With a reliability of 0.5, there is still a 37 per cent chance of reversal, a reliability of 0.8 will result in 20 per cent reversals, and 0.95 will result in their reversing order 2.2 per cent of the time. From this example, it is evident that reliability of 0.75 is a fairly minimal requirement for a useful instrument.

Improving reliability

If we return to the basic definition of reliability as a ratio of true variance between subjects to (true variance ± error variance), we can improve reliability only by increasing the magnitude of the variance between subjects relative to the error variance. This can be accomplished in a number of ways, both legitimate and illegitimate.

There are several approaches to reducing error variance. Many authors recommend observer training, although the specific strategies to be used in training raters are usually unspecified. Alternatively, Newble *et al.* (1980) have suggested that observers have difficulty acquiring new skills. They recommend, as a result, that if consistently extreme observers are discovered, they simply be eliminated from further use. The strategies for improving scale design discussed in Chapter 4 may also contribute to reducing error variance.

Similarly, there are a number of ways of enhancing the true variance. If the majority of individual scores are either very high or very low, so that the average score is approaching the maximum or minimum possible, then many of the items are being wasted. The solution is to introduce items that will result in performance nearer the middle of the scale, effectively increasing true variance. One could also modify the descriptions on the scale, for example by changing 'poor—fair—good—excellent' to 'fair—good—very good —excellent'.

An alternative approach, which is *not* legitimate, is to administer the test to a more heterogeneous group of subjects for the purpose of determining reliability. For example, if a measure of function in arthritis does not reliably discriminate among ambulatory arthritics, administering the test both to normal subjects and to bedridden hospitalized arthritics will almost certainly improve reliability. Of course the resulting reliability no longer yields any information about the ability of the instrument to discriminate among ambulatory patients.

By contrast, it is sometimes the case that a reliability coefficient derived from a homogeneous population is to be applied to a population which is more heterogeneous. It is clear from the above discussion that the reliability in the application envisioned will be larger than that determined in the homogeneous study population. If the standard deviations of the two samples are known, it is possible to calculate a new reliability coefficient, or to *correct for attenuation*, using the following formula:

$$R_{\text{revised}} = \frac{R \times \sigma^2_{\text{new}}}{R \times \sigma^2_{\text{new}} + (1 - R) \times \sigma^2_{\text{old}}}$$

where σ^2_{new} and σ^2_{old} are the variances of the new and original sample respectively, and R is the original reliability.

Perhaps the simplest way to improve reliability is to increase the number of items on the test. It is not self-evident why this should help, but the answer lies in statistical theory. As long as the test items are not perfectly correlated, the true variance will increase as the square of the number of items, whereas the error variance will increase only as the number of items. So if the test length is tripled, true variance will be nine times as large, and error variance three times as large as the original test. From the Spearman–Brown formula, which we discussed in Chapter 5, the new reliability will be:

$$R_{\text{SB}} = \frac{3 \times R}{1 + 2 \times R} \, .$$

So if the original reliability was 0.7, the tripled test will have a reliability of 0.875.

The Spearman–Brown formula can be used in another way. If we know the reliability of a test of a particular length is r and we wish to achieve a reliability of R, then the formula can be modified to indicate the factor by which we must increase the test length, k:

$$k = \frac{R\,(1 - r)}{r\,(1 - R)} \, .$$

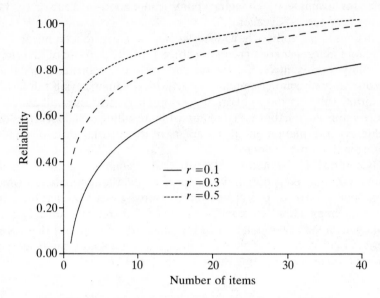

Fig. 8.3. Relation between number of items and reliability.

The relationship between the number of items and test length is shown in Figure 8.3.

To improve measures of stability, such as test–retest reliability, one can always shorten the retest interval. However, if the instrument is intended to measure states of duration of weeks or months, the demonstration of retest reliability over hours or days is not useful.

Finally, it is evident from the foregoing discussion that there is not a single reliability associated with a measure. A more useful approach to the issue of reliability is to critically examine the components of variance due to each source of variation in turn then focusing efforts on reducing the larger sources of error variance. This approach, called *generalizability theory*, is covered in the next chapter.

Different forms of the reliability coefficient

There has been considerable debate in the literature regarding which is the most appropriate choice of reliability coefficient. The coefficients we have derived in this chapter from ANOVA methods are all forms of 'intra-class correlation coefficients'. However, other methods, in particular the Pearson product-moment correlation and Cohen's Kappa (K) (Cohen 1960), are frequently recommended. Accordingly, we shall discuss these alternatives, and attempt to reconcile the differences among the measures.

Pearson correlation

The Pearson correlation is based on regression analysis, and is a measure of the extent to which the relationship between two variables can be described by a straight (regression) line. In the present context, this is a measure of the extent to which two observations on a group of subjects can be fitted by a straight line. One such relationship is shown in Figure 8.4. Note that a perfect fit is obtained, resulting in a Pearson correlation of 1.0 despite the fact that the intercept is non-zero and the slope is not equal to 1.0. By contrast, the intra-class correlation will yield a value of 1.0 only if all the observations on each subject are identical, which dictates a slope of 1.0 and intercept of 0.0. This suggests that the Pearson correlation is an inappropriate, and liberal measure of reliability; that is to say, the Pearson coefficient will usually be higher than the true reliability. In practice, however, the predominant source of error is usually due to random variation, and under these circumstances, the Pearson and intra-class correlations will be very close.

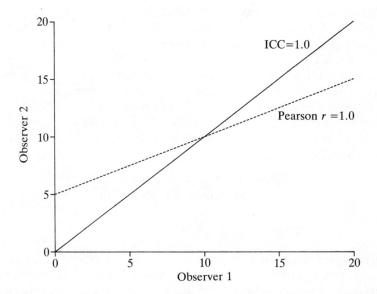

Fig. 8.4. Typical graph of inter-observer scores, showing difference between Pearson correlation and intra-class correlation.

Table 8.5   *Contingency table for two observers*

		Observer 2		
		Present	Absent	TOTAL
Observer	Present	20	15	35
1	Absent	10	55	65
	TOTAL	30	70	100

The K coefficient

At the beginning of this chapter, we gave an example where there were only two levels of measurement—presence or absence. We calculated a simple agreement as the proportion of responses in which the two observers agree. Although straightforward, this measure is very strongly influenced by the distribution of positives and negatives. If there is a preponderance of normal or abnormal cases, there will be a high agreement by chance alone. The *K* coefficient explicitly deals with this situation by examining the proportion of responses in the two agreement cells (yes/yes, no/no) in relation to the proportion of responses in these cells which would be expected by chance, given the marginal distributions.

For example, suppose we were to consider a judgement by two observers of the presence or absence of a Babinski sign (an upgoing toe following scratching of the bottom of the foot) on a series of neurological patients. The data might be displayed in a contingency table like Table 8.5.

The overall agreement is simply $(20 + 55)/100 = 0.75$. However, we would expect that a certain number of agreements would arise by chance alone. Specifically, we can calculate the expected agreement by chance from the marginals; the top left cell would have $(35 \times 30)/100 = 10.5$ expected, and the bottom right cell would have $(70 \times 65)/100 = 45.5$ expected, so that the expected proportion is $(10.5 + 45.5)/100$, or 0.555. The *K* coefficient corrects for chance agreement in the following manner:

$$K = \frac{(\text{observed proportion} - \text{expected proportion})}{1.0 - \text{expected proportion}}$$

$$= \frac{(0.75 - 0.555)}{(1.0 - 0.555)} = 0.43.$$

Therefore, instead of a raw agreement of .75, we end up with a chance-corrected agreement of .43. This effort may seem a little extreme. However, in circumstances where the frequency of positive results is very low, it is very easy to obtain impressive figures for agreement although agreement beyond chance is virtually absent.

In the example we have chosen, the approach to assessment of observer agreement appears to have little in common with our previous examples, where we used ANOVA methods. However, if we considered judgements which differ only slightly from Babinski signs, the parallel may become more obvious. For example, suppose the same observers were assessing muscle strength, which is conventionally done on a six-point scale from $0 =$ flaccid to $5 =$ normal strength. In this case a display of agreement would involve a 6×6 contingency table.

Since the coefficient we calculated previously considers only total agreement and does not provide partial credit for responses which differ by only one or two categories, it would be inappropriate for scaled responses as in the present example. However, an extension of the approach, called 'weighted K' (Cohen 1968), does consider partial agreement. Credit is given for partial agreement by assigning weights to the off-diagonal cells in such a manner that the top-left to bottom-right diagonal has weights of unity, and the opposite corners have weights of 0. As originally formulated, the weights could be assigned arbitrary values between 0 and 1. However, unless there are strong prior reasons, the most commonly used weighting scheme, called *quadratic weights*, which bases disagreement weights on the square of the amount of discrepancy, should be used. With quadratic weights, differences in one category are given a weight of 1, differences in two categories a weight of 4 (2^2) and so forth. *If this weighting scheme is used, then the weighted K is exactly identical to the intra-class correlation coefficient.* Conversely, a two-level response such as 'yes/no' can be coded as 0 and 1. If these numbers are analysed using ANOVA methods as in our original example, the resulting intraclass correlation will be identical to the unweighted K.

The discussion regarding appropriate measures of agreement is therefore easily resolved. The Pearson correlation is theoretically incorrect but usually fairly close. K and the intra-class correlation yield identical results, so the choice can be dictated by ease of calculation, nothing else.

References

Cohen, J. (1960). A coefficient of agreement for nominal scales. *Educational and Psychological Measurement*. **20**, 37–46.

Cohen, J. (1968). Weighted kappa: Nominal scale agreement with provision for scaled disagreement or partial credit. *Psychological Bulletin*, **70**, 213–20.

Guilford, J.P. (1956). *Psychometric methods*, (2nd edn.) McGraw Hill, New York.

Kelley, T.L. (1927). *Interpretation of educational measurements*. World Book, Yonkers.

Kline, P. (1986). *A handbook of test construction*. Methuen, London.

Newble, D.I., Hoare J., and Sheldrake, P.F. (1980). The selection and training of examiners for clinical examinations. *Medical Education*, **4**, 345–9.

Nunnally, J.C. (1978). *Psychometric theory*. McGraw–Hill, New York.

Thorndike, R.L. and Hagen, E. (1969). *Measurement and evaluation in education and psychology*. Wiley, New York.

Weiner, E.A. and Stewart, B.J. (1984). *Assessing individuals*. Little Brown, Boston.

9

Generalizability theory

Classical test theory, upon which the reliability coefficient is based, begins with a simple assumption—that an observed test score can be decomposed into a 'true' score (which no one really knows!) and an 'error' score. This assumption then leads directly to the formulation of the reliability coefficient as the ratio of true variance to (true + error) variance, as discussed in the previous chapter.

We saw that there are many approaches to estimating reliability, each of which generates a different coefficient. One can examine scores from the same observer on two viewings of the same stimulus (intra-observer), different observers (inter-observer), different occasions separated by a short time interval (test–retest), different forms of the scale (parallel forms) and so on. Further, these standard measures do not exhaust the possible sources of variance. For example, measures such as bone density or tenderness might be expected to be equal on both sides of the body (left–right reliability?). Skin colour might be expected to be the same on the soles of hands and feet (top–bottom reliability?).

Clearly, the assumption that all variance in scores can be neatly divided into true and error variance is simplistic. Instead, for each person we have measured, our goal is to obtain the most precise estimate we can of the score that person should have if there were no sources of error contaminating our results. One way to think about it is the following.

Imagine that we could identify all the likely sources of error in a measurement of some characteristic of a person. Having made this step, e.g. declaring that the important sources of error in this measurement situation were the observer, the time of day, and the form of the test (interview, telephone or self-administered), we have then defined our 'universe' of possible observations to include different observers, morning, noon, and night, and three test forms. If we then proceeded to average each person's scores over all these possible conditions, this would be an unbiased estimate of that person's score over the universe as we have defined it. Note that there is no pretence that this is a 'true' score, since we may well have guessed wrong about the universe—maybe the phases of Mars really mattered—but this is still a best guess at a 'universe' score for our predefined universe of observations.

The next step would be to use the data we have gathered to determine the extent to which each of these variables actually influenced the score. For example, if scores were always higher on a telephone interview, or if some people scored higher in a face-to-face interview, then we must be concerned that test format is contributing some variability to any observed score.

One way of expressing this variability is to use ANOVA concepts, as we did in Chapter 8. Thus, to the extent that the phase of the moon does influence the obtained scores, then the analysis of the data will show that the variance due to lunar phase will be large relative to other components. Conversely, if the sources we have identified are not important, and we have missed some important sources of error, then there will be a large amount of variance due to 'random error' or 'residual'. By identifying these sources of error, we can determine the relative importance of each component in adding error to a measurement. In turn, this information can then lead to specific strategies to reduce major components of error and improve measurement, the details of which will be discussed later.

It is evident that the conventional approaches to reliability: test—retest, inter-observer, and so on, become simply special cases of a more general formulation which seeks to identify the important sources of variance in a particular measurement situation from the outset, and then attempt to quantify these sources of error.

This broad approach was originally devised by Cronbach *et al.* (1972) and is known as *generalizability theory*. The essence of the theory is the recognition that in any measurement situation there are multiple (in fact infinite) sources of variance (called *facets* in the theory). An important goal of measurement is to attempt to identify and measure variance components which are contributing error to an estimate, and then implement strategies to reduce the influence of these sources on the measurement. Although there have been relatively few applications of generalizability theory in medicine (Boodoo and O'Sullivan 1982; Chambers *et al.* 1987; Evans *et al.* 1981), the method is an elegant and practical way to approach issues of reliability, and more applications will probably emerge in future.

An example

An example may clarify the theory. Imagine a group of respiratory patients enrolled in a rehabilitation program. In order to determine the reliability of measurement of pulmonary function, three physiotherapists make independent assessments on two successive visits 5 days apart. The design may look like Table 9.1.

It is evident that this design contains elements of both inter-observer and

Table 9.1 *Assessment of ten patients by three physiotherapists on two days*

Patient	Observer 1		Observer 2		Observer 3	
	Day 1	Day 5	Day 1	Day 5	Day 1	Day 5
1						
2						
.						
.						
.						
10						

Experimental Design

test–retest reliability. To the extent that the scores assigned by different therapists on the same day differ, this will contribute to a reduction in inter-observer reliability. Observations by the *same* observer on the second occasion are a measure of test–retest reliability.

What makes this design approach different from conventional assessment is that both sources of error (therapist and occasion) are incorporated in the *same* design, instead of conducting two separate studies. This approach has two methodological advantages: first, the estimate of each reliability is derived from multiple observations, since three raters are contributing to the assessment of test–retest reliability and two occasions are summed together to yield a measure of inter-observer reliability. This effectively increases the sample size and thereby improves precision. Second, the combining of the two sources of variation into one experiment permits the consideration of additional combinations of error variance. For example, it is likely that our real concern is the reliability of an observation made by *any* therapist on *any* occasion; a situation which would suggest the need for a test–retest—inter-observer reliability coefficient. This coefficient can be easily determined from a design such as that in the example, but would not normally be available from applications of classical test theory.

G Studies

In practice, we would be unlikely to stop at just two sources of variation if we were serious about applying concepts of generalizability. For example, there is some evidence that the encouragement provided by the therapist may affect performance on pulmonary function tests, suggesting that it would be worth investigating the effect of therapists offering high or low levels of encouragement. We might wish to explore other variables such as the effect of time of day, or the familiarity of the patient with the therapist by systematically varying these factors. The broad approach is referred to as a generalizability study, or '*G study*'.

It is evident that the number of variables to include in the design is limited only by the imagination of the investigator and the time and stamina of the observers. Of course there are logistical, and as it turns out, methodological constraints on the number of variables which can be included in the design. Nevertheless, the intent of this study is to identify all the major potential sources of variation so that the variance attributed to each source relative to each other can be determined.

D studies

Having conducted such a study, the users of the instrument are then in a position to determine the generalizability coefficient appropriate for their particular circumstances. Further, once the components of variance are identified, we can explore how the reliability would change if we took certain decisions. For example, we might contrast the effect of using the average score of four raters, which would lower the variance components associated with raters by a factor of 2, against the impact of averaging scores obtained under both high and low encouragement conditions, which would reduce the variance components associated with encouragement by a factor of 2. These explorations of the impact of certain decision rules are called decision studies, or '*D studies*'.

Continuing with the example, we might explore how the various components of variance are derived. For simplicity, we limit ourselves to the two-factor case, including only variation due to multiple observers and repeated occasions of observation. If these data were analysed using repeated-measures ANOVA, the resulting table would resemble Table 9.2.

Note that this table includes the expected mean squares, expressed as a sum of variance components. The detailed derivation of these expressions can be found in statistics texts (e.g. Glass and Stanley 1970), so we just give a brief indication of the conceptual basis of the expressions.

The basic notion of the mean square (MS) as a sum of variances was discussed in Chapter 8. Every MS contains both the variance due to the factor of interest and also variance due to all other sources which interact with it; so for example, the MS due to observers contains variance due to observers, and also variance due to the interaction between observers and patients, observers and days, and observers, days and patients (which is just the residual error term in this example). At first sight, this seems non-

Table 9.2 *Analysis of variance table*

Source	Sum of squares	d.f.	Mean square (MS)	Expected mean square (EMS)
Patients (p)	3915	9	435	$\sigma^2_{dop} + 2\sigma^2_{op} + 3\sigma^2_{dp} + 6\sigma^2_p$
Day (d)	815	1	815	$\sigma^2_{dop} + 3\sigma^2_{dp} + 10\sigma^2_{do} + 30\sigma^2_d$
Day × Patients (dp)	585	9	65	$\sigma^2_{dop} + 3\sigma^2_{dp}$
Observer (o)	960	2	480	$\sigma^2_{dop} + 2\sigma^2_{op} + 10\sigma^2_{do} + 20\sigma^2_o$
Observer × Patients (op)	540	18	30	$\sigma^2_{dop} + 2\sigma^2_{op}$
Day × Observer (do)	340	2	170	$\sigma^2_{dop} + 10\sigma^2_{do}$
Day × Observer × Patients (dop)	360	18	20	σ^2_{dop}

sensical, since we have already separately calculated the variance due to all these other interactions. However, the apparent contradiction resides in the basic assumption of statistics which distinguishes between samples and populations. The MS terms we have calculated are *estimates* of the population variances, expressed in σ^2 terms. Even if, for example, there really was no overall difference between observers, or no 'main effect' of observers, we might expect that random fluctuations would result in some difference between the calculated means for each observer, and hence some non-zero value of the MS due to observers. The extent to which this calculated MS differs from the population variance due to observers is imbedded in the magnitude of the interaction terms, thus these interactions contribute to the expected MS.

Furthermore, each MS is actually summed up over all levels of the factors *not* contained in the expression; the dp interaction is summed over the three levels of the observer, and the o main effect is summed over the ten levels of patients and two levels of days. As a result, when these variance components are entered into the expected mean square (EMS) expression, they contain multipliers accounting for the levels of the factors *not* in each term.

Further elaboration of the derivation of these expressions is beyond the scope of this book. Suffice it say that from these formulae we can derive the resulting variance components. These are shown below Table 9.3.

Table 9.3   *Components of variance*

Source	Variance
Patients	60
Day	20
Day × Patients	15
Observer	15
Observer × Patients	5
Day × Observer	15
Day × Observer × Patients	20

From this analysis, it is apparent that the main source of variance in the measurements is p, which indicates that most of the variability in the measurements is due to systematic differences between patients. This is the expectation, and indicates that we were successful in discriminating among patients. Relatively less variance is due to the main effects of d (suggesting systematically higher or lower values in different days) and o (reflecting systematic differences between observers). The dp interaction shows that some patients did better on Day 1 than Day 5, while this was reversed for other patients. The od interaction is interpreted in a similar manner. The low variance due to the op interaction is encouraging, reflecting that the observers' ratings are *not* influenced by specific patients. Finally, the residual (dop) interaction is moderately large (20) in comparison to the remaining sources of variance, possibly suggesting that there are other important factors we might have included in the *G* study.

Applying the approaches of the previous chapter, we could easily conjure up a reliability coefficient consisting of the variance due to patients (60), divided by the sum of all the variance components (150), or 0.4. Unfortunately, this approach simply indicates that the other factors are contributing considerable error variance, but does not indicate where it came from or how one might improve the situation.

Let us examine Table 9.3 in more detail. First, note that the main effects of d and o imply simply that the average score on Day 1 differed from the score on Day 5, and that there were differences in the average scores of the observers. This may be of no consequence if we simply wish to compare scores on the same day or by the same observer, or alternatively if we are willing to apply a correction factor to eliminate this source of bias in each estimate. Conversely, the interaction terms between p and the other variables represent the extent to which each source directly contributes *random* variation to a score. For example, the op interaction implies that some patients are rated differently by some observers than by other observers, an effect that we cannot disentangle if we wish to use scores obtained from different observers. However, this interaction term is irrelevant if we wish to look only at reliability of the ratings by the same observer on successive days. In this case, the dp interaction term expresses the amount of random error in repeated scores by the same observer.

These observations suggest that it may be possible to use the variance components identified in the analysis of variance to construct a series of coefficients which will depend on the variables which will remain constant (or 'fixed') in a particular measurement situation, and the variables one wishes to make generalizations over.

Continuing with this example, suppose we want to use these data to examine inter-observer reliability. In this case, the fact that the observations were repeated on two occasions is incidental; what we want to focus on is differences between observers. The design looks as if we had done an inter-observer reliability study twice.

In examining inter-observer reliability, then, the change in scores that occurred with the passage of time is incidental, and so the main effect of 'day' would be excluded from the sources of variance in this generalizability coefficient. Second, if the 'day' factor were not explicitly calculated as a variance component, then the interaction between 'day' and 'patients' factor would end up in the sum of squares due to 'patients'. So if we wish to calculate the coefficient equivalent to an inter-observer reliability, the numerator would contain the main effect of 'patients', and the interaction between 'patients' and 'day'.

Extrapolating from this example, then, in constructing a generalizability coefficient, the numerator of the coefficient contains the variance due to patients and all interactions between patients and any factors over which one does not wish to generalize (such as day). The denominator contains variance due to patients, interactions between patients and all other factors, and the random error term (in this case, patient × observer × time). The generalizability coefficient becomes:

$$\frac{\sigma^2_p + \sigma^2_{dp}}{\sigma^2_p + \sigma^2_{op} + \sigma^2_{dp} + \sigma^2_{dop}} = \frac{60 + 15}{60 + 5 + 15 + 20} = 0.75.$$

In looking at the test–retest reliability, the opposite situation arises. In this circumstance, variance due to systematic differences between observers (i.e. the main effect of o) is irrelevant. Analogously, the op interaction is incorporated into the variance due to patients in the numerator of the coefficient. So the generalizability coefficient becomes:

$$\frac{\sigma^2_p + \sigma^2_{op}}{\sigma^2_p + \sigma_{2op} + \sigma^2_{dp} + \sigma^2_{dop}} = \frac{60 + 5}{60 + 5 + 15 + 20} = 0.65.$$

Finally, one may wish to generalize from an observation by one observer on one day to an observation by a different observer at another time. This coefficient has no classical equivalent, and equals

$$\frac{\sigma^2_p}{\sigma^2_p + \sigma^2_{op} + \sigma^2_{dp} + \sigma^2_{dop}} = \frac{60}{60 + 5 + 15 + 20} = 0.60.$$

As one would expect, this coefficient is lower than either of the preceding coefficients.

This example provides some insight into the nature of generalizability theory. The approach begins by attempting to define all the significant sources of observational error—observers, days, items, etc. These are then incorporated into a factorial experimental design, and components of variance determined. Different coefficients can then be calculated depending on which factors ('facets' in the theory) will remain fixed, and which will vary.

The example we used was based in a simple ANOVA design, in which there were two factors, and each factor occurred at all levels of the other factors, a 'crossed' design in the language of analysis of variance. However, the method can be used with more complex designs, including as many as four or five factors, and including 'nested' designs, where the factor structure is more complex. The general approach remains the same; to begin by isolating the various sources of variance in the scores, and then generate a family of coefficients which depend on the particular factors which are allowed to vary and remain fixed.

D Study application

Generalizabilty theory has several advantages over classical approaches. Since efforts were made to explicitly identify components of variance, we are now in a position to investigate strategies to reduce error. The impact of various decisions on reliability can be explicitly determined, and is pursued in the context of what has been called a *D* study.

For example, we noted in our previous example that the observer was a relatively small source of variance compared to the day of assessment. Therefore, one appropriate strategy would be to take assessments on several days using a single observer. The alternative strategy of gathering several observations from multiple observers on a single day would provide relatively little gain.

The effect of these strategies can be quantified in the following manner. Since the variance of the average of *n* observations is just the initial variance divided by *n*, this can be included in the generalizability coefficients. Compare two strategies:

(1) one observer on three successive days;
(2) four observers on a single day.

For case (1), the variance due to dp and the error variance will be reduced by a factor of 3, so the new coefficient is

$$G = \frac{60}{60 + 5 + 15/3 + 20/3} = 0.78.$$

Similarly, the coefficient for the second strategy will have the op interaction and the error variance divided by 4, to result in

$$G = \frac{60}{60 + 5/4 + 15 + 20/4} = 0.74.$$

Therefore the second strategy resulted in a lower coefficient, even though it involved one extra observation.

Summary

Although generalizability theory is difficult to comprehend, the value of the methods lies in the reinterpretation of the nature of measurement afforded by the theory. Instead of conceptualizing a measurement as a sum of a 'true' score and an 'error' score, generalizability theory forces a critical examination of the *sources* of measurement error. In addition, the effect of particular strategies to reduce error, based on multiple observations, can be directly estimated. As a result, the theory represents a powerful tool in advancing the methods of measurement.

References

Boodoo, G. M., and O'Sullivan, P. (1982). Obtaining generalizability coefficients for clinical evaluations. *Evaluation and the Health Professions*, **5**, 345–58.

Chambers, L. W., Haight, M., Norman, G. R., and MacDonald, L. (1987). Effect of mode of administration on a health status measure's responsiveness to change. *Medical Care*, **25**, 470–80.

Cronbach, L. J., Gleser, G. C., Nanda, H., and Rajaratnam, N. (1972). *The dependability of behavioral measurements: Theory of generalizability for scores and profiles*. Wiley, New York.

Evans, W. J., Cayten, C. G., and Green, P. A. (1981). Determining the generalizability of rating scales in clinical settings. *Medical Care*, **19**, 1211–19.

Glass, G. V., and Stanley, J. C. (1970). *Statistical methods in education and psychology*. Prentice-Hall, Englewood Cliffs, NJ.

10

Validity

In the previous chapters, we examined various aspects of reliability; that is, how reproducible the results of a scale are under different conditions. This is a necessary step in establishing the usefulness of a measure, but it is not sufficient. The next step is to determine if the scale is measuring what we think it is; that is, the scale's *validity*. To illustrate the difference, imagine that we are trying to develop a new index to measure the degree of headache pain. We find that patients get the same score when they are tested on two different occasions, that different interviewers get similar results when assessing the same patient, and so on; in other words, the index is reliable. However, we still have no proof that differences in the total score reflect the degree of headache pain: the scale may be measuring pain from other sources; or it may be tapping factors entirely unrelated to pain, such as depression or the tendency to complain of bodily ailments. In this chapter, we will examine how to determine if we can draw valid conclusions from the scale.

Why assess validity?

The question that immediately arises is why we have to establish validity in the first place. After all, the health care fields are replete with measures that have never been 'validated' through any laborious testing process. Despite this, no one questions the usefulness of taking a patient's temperature to detect the presence of fever, or of keeping track of the height and weight of an infant to check growth, or getting T4 levels on people with suspected thyroid problems. Why, then, are there a multitude of articles addressing the problems of trying to test for validity? There are two answers to this question: the nature of *what* is being measured; and the *relationship* of that variable to its purported cause.

Many variables measured in the health sciences are physical quantities, such as height, serum cholesterol level, or BUN. As such, they are readily observable, either directly or with the correct instruments. Irrespective of who manufactured the thermometer, different nurses will get the same reading, within the limits of reliability discussed in Chapters 8 and 9. Moreover, there is little question that what is being measured is temperature; no one would state that the height of the mercury in the tube is really due to something else, like blood pressure or pH level.

The situation is different when we turn to variables like 'range of motion', 'quality of life', or 'responsibility as a physician'. As we discuss later in this chapter, the measurements of these factors are dependent upon their definitions, which may vary from one person to another, and the way they are measured. For example, some theorists hold that 'social support' can be assessed by counting the number of people a person has contact with during a fixed period of time. Other theories state that the person's perceptions of who is available in times of need are more important; while yet another school of thought is that the reciprocity of the helping relationship is crucial. Since social support is not something which can be observed and measured directly, various questionnaires have been developed to assess it, each reflecting a different underlying theory. Needless to say, each instrument yields a somewhat different result, raising the question of which, if any, gives the 'correct' answer.

The second reason why validity testing is required in some areas but not others depends on the relationship between the observation and what it reflects. Based on years of observation or our knowledge of how the body works, the validity of a test may be self-evident. For instance, since the kidneys regulate the level of sodium in the body, it makes sense to measure urine sodium to determine the presence of renal disease. On the other hand, we do not know ahead of time whether a physiotherapist's evaluations of patients' level of functioning bear any relationship to their actual performance once they are discharged from hospital. Similarly, we may hypothesize that students who have spent time doing volunteer work for service agencies will make better physicians or nurses. However, since our knowledge of the determinants of human behaviour is far from perfect, this prediction will have to be validated against actual performance.

The 'types' of validity

One of the most difficult aspects of validity testing is the terminology. Until the 1970s, almost all textbooks adopted a 'trinitarian' point of view (Landy 1986), dividing this topic into the 'three Cs' of *content* validity, *criterion* validity, and *construct* validity (terms we will discuss later). These were seen as three relatively separate attributes of a measure which had to be independently established. More recently, though, two seemingly different trends have emerged. First, a proliferation of new 'types' of validity were proposed. For example, construct validity was differentiated into various classes such as trait validity, discriminant validity, convergent validity, and so forth (see, for example, Messick 1980). At the same time, a second trend led to a reconceptualization of the process of validity testing itself and what could actually be concluded from a demonstration of validity in one form or another.

Previously, testing for validity was seen as demonstrating the psychometric properties of a *scale*. Led by Cronbach (1971), though, the focus changed to emphasize the characteristics of the *people* who are assessed. As Landy (1986) puts it, 'Validation processes are not so much directed toward the integrity of tests as they are directed toward the inferences that can be made about the attributes of the people who have produced those test scores' (p. 1186). In other words, validating a scale is really a process whereby we determine the degree of confidence we can place on inferences we make about people based on their scores from that scale.

Seen from this perspective, the two trends are actually just different aspects of the same thing. Validation is a process of *hypothesis testing*: 'Someone who scores high on this measure will also do well in situation A, perform poorly on test B, and will differ from those who score low on the scale on traits C and D.' So, rather than being constrained by the trinitarian Cs mentioned above, scale constructors are limited only by their imagination in devising experiments to test their hypotheses. In the past, students (and their teachers) have spent much time arguing whether a specific study demonstrated, for example, criterion or construct validity. Now, the important questions are, 'Does the hypothesis of this validation study make sense in light of what the scale is designed to measure', and 'Do the results of this study allow us to draw the inferences that we wish to make?'

Unfortunately, this creates difficulties for writers of textbooks. From the new perspective, a chapter on validity would focus primarily on the logic and methodology of hypothesis testing. The student, though, will continue to encounter terms like 'construct validity' and 'criterion validity' in his or her readings for some time to come. We have chosen here to take the middle ground; to organize the chapter around the traditional headings, but at the same time to emphasize that rather than being disparate attributes, the various 'types' of validity are all addressing the same issue of the degree of confidence we can place in the inferences we draw from scores on scales.

Content validity

We mentioned content validity previously within the context of issues surrounding item construction (Chapter 3). Here, let us briefly touch on it again from our new vantage point. When we conclude that a student has 'passed' a test in, say, respirology, or that an arthritic patient has a grip strength of only 10 kg, we are making the assumption that the measures comprise representative samples of the disorders, behaviours, attitudes, or knowledge that we want to assess. That is, we do not too much care if the student knows the specific bits of information tapped by the examination, or how much the patient can squeeze a dynamometer. Going back to what validity testing is all about, our aim is *inferential*; a person who does well on the exam can be expected to know more about lungs than a student who does poorly, and a patient who has a weaker grip has more severe arthritis than someone who can exert more pressure.

A measure that includes a more representative sample of the target behaviour lends itself to more accurate inferences; that is, inferences which hold true under a wider range of circumstances. If there are important aspects of the outcome that are missed by the scales, then we are likely to make some inferences which will prove to be wrong; our *inferences* (not the instruments) are invalid. For example, if there was nothing on the respirology examination regarding oxygen exchange, then it is quite possible that a high scorer on the test may *not* know more about this topic than a student with a lower score. Similarly, grip strength has relatively poor content validity; as such, it does not allow us to make accurate inferences about other attributes of the rheumatoid patient, such as erythrocyte sedimentation rate, joint count, or morning stiffness, except insofar as these indices are correlated with grip strength.

Thus, the higher the content validity of a measure, the broader are the inferences that we can validly draw about the person under a variety of conditions and in different situations.

We discussed in previous chapters that reliability places an upper limit on validity, so that the higher the reliability, the higher the maximum possible validity (more formally, the maximum validity of a test is the square root of reliability coefficient). There is one notable exception to this general rule: the relationship between internal consistency (an index of reliability) and content validity. If we are tapping a behaviour, disorder, or trait that is relatively heterogeneous, like rheumatoid arthritis, then it is quite conceivable that the scale will have low internal consistency; not all patients with a high joint count have a high sedimentation rates or morning stiffness. We could increase the internal consistency of the index by eliminating items which are not highly correlated with each other or the total score. If we did this, though, we would end up with an index tapping only one aspect of arthritis—stiffness, for example—and which therefore has very low content validity. Under such circumstances, it is better to sacrifice internal consistency for content validity. The ultimate aim of the scale is inferential, which depends more on content validity than internal consistency.

Criterion validity

The traditional definition of criterion validity is the correlation of a scale with some other measure of the trait or disorder under study, ideally, a 'gold standard' which has been used and accepted in the field. Criterion validity is usually divided into two types: *concurrent* validity and *predictive* validity. With concurrent validity, we correlate the new scale with the criterion measure, both of which are given at the same time. For example, we could administer a new scale for depression and the Beck Depression Inventory (an accepted measure of depression) during the same interview, or within a short time of each other. In predictive validity, the criterion will not be available until some time in the future. The major areas where this latter form of criterion validity is used are in college admission tests, where the ultimate outcome is the person's performance on graduation four years hence; or diagnostic tests, where we must await the outcome of an autopsy or the further progression of the disease to confirm or disconfirm our predictions.

A major question is why, if a good criterion measure already exists, are we going through the often laborious process of developing a new instrument? Leaving aside the unworthy (if prevalent) reasons of trying to cash in on a lucrative market, or having an instrument with one's name as part of the title, there are a number of valid reasons. The existing test can be expensive, invasive, dangerous, or time-consuming; or the outcome may not be known until it is too late. The first three reasons are the usual rationales for scales which require concurrent validation, and the last reason for those which need predictive validity. On the basis of these reasons for developing new tests, Messick (1980) has proposed using the terms *diagnostic utility* or *substitutability* for concurrent validity, and *predictive utility* for predictive validity; while they are not yet widely used, these are far more descriptive terms for the rationales underlying criterion validity testing.

As an example of the use of concurrent validity, let us look at the usual standard test for tuberculosis, the chest X-ray. While it is still used as the definitive criterion, it suffers from a number of drawbacks which make it a less than ideal test, especially for routine screening. It is somewhat invasive—exposing the patient to low levels of ionizing radiation, and expensive—requiring a costly machine, film, a trained technician, and a radiologist to interpret the results. For these reasons, it would be desirable to develop a cheaper and less risky test for screening purposes. This new tool would then be compared, in a concurrent validation study, to the chest X-ray.

Within the realm of predictive validity, we would like to know *before* students are admitted to graduate or professional school whether or not

Table 10.1 *Fourfold table to evaluate criterion validity for scales with dichotomous outcomes*

X-ray results

	TB	No TB
TB	a	b
No TB	c	d

Mantoux test

they will graduate four years later, rather than having to incur the expense of the training and possibly denying admission to someone who will do well. So, administering our scale prior to admission, we would determine how well it predicts graduate status or performance on a licensing examination.

Let us go through the usual procedures for establishing these two forms of validity and their rationales. As we have mentioned, the most commonly used design for concurrent validity is to administer the new scale and the standard at the same time. Staying with the example of a new test for TB, we would give both the Mantoux test (assuming it is the one being validated) and the X-ray to a large group of people. Since the outcome is dichotomous (the person either has or does not have abnormalities on the X-ray consistent with TB), we would draw up a fourfold table, as in Table 10.1.

We could analyse the results using either the indices of sensitivity and specificity, or some measure of correlation which can be derived from a 2 × 2 table, such as the phi coefficient (ϕ). This coefficient is related to χ^2 by the formula

$$\phi = \sqrt{\frac{\chi^2}{N}} ,$$

or can be calculated from Table 10.1 using the equation

$$\phi = \frac{BC - AD}{\sqrt{[(A + B) (C + D) (A + C) (B + D)]}}$$

If our measures were continuous, as would be found if we were validating a new measure of depression against the *Beck Depression Inventory* or

CES-D (another accepted index of depression), we would use a Pearson correlation coefficient. In either case, we would be looking for a strong association between our new measure and the already existing one. This would indicate that a person who has a high score or comes out 'diseased' on the new test would be expected to have a high score (or have been labelled as diseased) on the more established instrument.

In assessing predictive validity, the person is given the new measure at Time 1, and then the standard some time later, at Time 2. Again, we would use a fourfold table to evaluate a scale with a dichotomous outcome, and a correlational measure if the outcome were continuous. However, there is one additional point which appears obvious, but is often overlooked; *no decision can be made based on the new instrument*. For example, if we were trying to establish the validity of an autobiographical letter as a criterion for admission to medical or nursing school, we would have all applicants write these missives. Then, no matter how good we felt this measure was, we would immediately put the evaluations of the letters in a safe place, without looking at them, and base our decisions on other criteria. Only after the students had or had not graduated would we take out the scores, and compare them with actual performance.

What would happen if we violated this proscription, and used the letters to help us decide who should be admitted? We would be able to determine what proportion of students who wrote excellent letters graduated four years later (cell A in Table 10.1) and what proportion failed (cell B). However, we would *not* be able to state what proportion of those who wrote 'poor' letters would have gone on to pass with flying colours (cell C), nor how good letters are in detecting people who will fail (cell D): they would never be given the chance. In this case, the sample has been *truncated* on the basis of our new test and, as we will describe later in more detail, the correlation between our new test and the standard will be reduced, perhaps significantly.

A somewhat different situation can also occur with diagnostic tests. If the final diagnosis (the gold standard) were predicated in part on the results of our new instrument, then we have artificially built in a high correlation between the two; we are correlating the new measure with an outcome based on it. For example, in the process of validating two-dimensional echo-cardiography for diagnosing mitral valve prolapse (MVP), we would use the clinician's judgement of the presence or absence of MVP as the criterion. However, the clinician may know the results of the echo tests, and temper his diagnosis in light of them. This differs from our previous example in that we have not truncated our sample; rather, we are indirectly using the results of our new scale in both the predictor and the outcome. The technical term for this is *criterion contamination*.

In summary, then, criterion validity assesses how a person who scores at a certain level on our new scale does on some criterion measure. The usual experimental design is a correlational one; both measures are taken on a series of individuals. In the case of concurrent validity, the two results are gathered close together in time. In predictive validity, the results from the criterion measure are usually not known for some time, which can be between a few days to a few years later.

Construct validity

What is construct validity?

Attributes such as height or weight are readily observable, or can be 'operationally defined'; that is, defined by the way they are measured. Systolic blood pressure, for example, is the amount of pressure, measured in millimetres of mercury, at the moment of ventricular systole. Once we move away from the realm of physical attributes into more 'psychological' ones like anxiety, intelligence, or pain, however, we begin dealing with more abstract variables, ones that cannot be directly observed. We cannot 'see' anxiety; all we can observe are behaviours which, according to our theory of anxiety, are the results of it. We would attribute the sweaty palms, tachycardia, pacing back and forth, and difficulty in concentrating experienced by a student just prior to writing an exam, to his or her anxiety. Similarly, we may have two patients who, to all intents and purposes, have the same degree of angina. One patient has quit his job and spends most of the day sitting in a chair; the other continues working and is determined to 'fight it'. We may explain these differences in terms of such attitudes as 'motivation', 'illness behaviour', or the 'sick role model'. Again, these factors are not seen directly, only their hypothesized manifestations in terms of the patients' observable behaviours.

These proposed underlying factors are referred to as *hypothetical constructs*, or, more simply as *constructs*. A construct can be thought of as a 'mini-theory' to explain the relationships among various behaviours or attitudes. Many constructs arose from larger theories or clinical observations, before there were any ways of objectively measuring their effects. This would include terms like 'anxiety' or 'repression', derived from psychoanalytic theory; or 'sick role behaviour', which was based mainly on sociological theorizing. Other concepts, like the difference between 'fluid' and 'crystallized' intelligence (Cattell 1963), were proposed to explain observed correlations among variables which were already measured with a high degree of reliability.

It is fair to say that most psychological instruments and many measures of health are designed to tap some aspect of a hypothetical construct.

There are two reasons for wanting to develop such an instrument: the construct is a new one, and no scale exists which measures it; or we are dissatisfied with the existing tools, and feel that they omit some key aspect of the construct. Note that we are doing more than replacing one tool with a shorter, cheaper, or less invasive one, which is the rationale for criterion validity. Rather, we are using the underlying theory to help us develop a new or better instrument, where 'better' means able to explain a broader range of findings, explain them in a more parsimonious manner, or make more accurate predictions about a person's behaviour.

Establishing construct validity

As an example, consider the quest to develop a short checklist or scale to identify patients with irritable bowel syndrome (IBS). First, though, we should address the issue of why we consider IBS to be a construct rather than a disease like ulcers or amoebic dysentery. The central issue is that we cannot (at least not yet) definitively prove that a person has IBS; it is diagnosed by excluding other possible causes of the patient's symptoms. There is no X-ray or laboratory test to which we can point and say, 'Yes, that person has IBS'. Moreover, there is no known pathogen which produces the constellation of symptoms. We tie them together conceptually by postulating an underlying disorder which cannot be measured directly, in much the same way that we say a large vocabulary, a breadth of knowledge, and skill at problem-solving are all outward manifestations of a postulated but unseen concept we label 'intelligence'. Many of what physicians call 'syndromes' would be called 'hypothetical constructs' by psychologists and test developers. Indeed, even some 'diseases' like schizophrenia, Alzheimer's, or systemic lupus erythematosus, are closer to constructs than actual entities, since their diagnosis is based on constellations of symptoms, and there are no unequivocal diagnostic tests which can be used with living patients. This is more than just semantics, though. It implies that tests for diagnosing or measuring syndromes should be constructed in an analogous manner to those for more 'psychological' attributes.

The first indices developed for assessing IBS consisted, in the main, of two parts: exclusion of other diseases, and the presence of some physical signs and symptoms like pain in the lower left quadrant and diarrhoea without pain. These scales proved to be inadequate, as many patients 'diagnosed' by them were later discovered to have stomach cancer or other diseases, and patients who were missed were, a few years later, indistinguishable from IBS patients. Thus, new scales were developed which added other—primarily demographic and personality—factors, predicated on a broader view (a revised construct) of IBS, as a disorder marked by specific demography and a unique psychological configuration, in addition to the physical symptoms. The problem the test developers now faced was how to demonstrate that the new index was better than the older ones.

To address this problem, let us go back to what we mean by a 'valid' scale: it is one that allows us to make accurate inferences about a person. These inferences are derived from the construct, and are of the form; 'Based on my theory of construct X, people who score high on a test of X differ from people who score low on it in terms of attributes A, B, and C', where A, B, and C can be other instruments, behaviours, diagnoses, and so on. In this particular case, we would say, 'Based on my concept of IBS, high scorers on the index should (a) have symptoms which will not clear with conventional therapy, and (b) have a lower prevalence of organic bowel disease on autopsy.'

Since we are testing constructs, this form of testing is called *construct validation*. Methodologically, it differs from the types of validity testing we discussed previously in a number of important ways. First, content and criterion validity can often be established with one or two studies. However, we are often able to make many different predictions based on our theory or construct. For example, if we were validating a new scale of anxiety, just a few of the many hypotheses we can derive would be, 'Anxious people would have more rapid heart rates during an exam than low anxious ones'; 'Anxious people should do better on simple tasks than non-anxious subjects, but poorer than them on complex tasks'; or 'If I artificially induce anxiety with some experimental manoeuvre, then the subjects should score higher on my test'.

Thus, there is no one single experiment which can unequivocally 'prove' a construct. Construct validation is an on-going process, of learning more about the construct, making new predictions, and then testing them. Albert Einstein once said that there have been hundreds of experiments supporting his theory of relativity, but it would take only one non-confirmatory study to disprove it. So it is with construct validation; each supportive study serves only to strengthen what Cronbach and Meehl (1955) call the 'nomological network' of the interlocking predictions of a theory, but a single, well-designed experiment with negative findings can call into question the entire construct.

A second major difference between construct validity and the other types is that, with the former, we are assessing both the theory and the measure at the same time. Returning to our example of a better index for IBS, one prediction was that patients who have a high score would not respond to conventional therapy. Assume that we gave the index to a sample of patients presenting at a gastrointestinal (GI) clinic, and gave them all regular treatment. (Remember, we cannot base any decisions on the results of a scale we are validating; this would lead to criterion contamination.) If it turned out that our prediction were confirmed, then it would

lend credence to both our concept of IBS and the index we developed to measure it. However, if high-scoring subjects responded to treatment in about the same proportion as low scorers, then the problem could be that:
- our instrument is good, but the theory is wrong,
- the theory is fine, but our index cannot discriminate between IBS patients and those with other GI problems, or
- both the theory is wrong and our scale is useless.

Moreover, we would have no way of knowing which of these situations obtains until we do more studies.

A further complication enters the picture when we use an experimental study to validate the scale. Using the example of a new measure of anxiety, one prediction was that if we artificially induce anxiety, as in threatening the subject with an electric shock if he or she performs poorly on some task, then we should see an increase in scores on the index. If the scores do not go up, then the problem could be in either of the areas already mentioned—the theory and the measure—plus one other; both the theory and the scale are fine, but the experiment did not induce anxiety, as we had hoped it would. Again, any combination of these problems could be working: the measure is valid and the experiment worked, but the theory is wrong; the theory is right and the experiment went the way we planned, but the index is not measuring anxiety; and so forth.

We said that construct validity differs from content and criterion validity methodologically. At the risk of being repetitive, we should emphasize that construct validation does not *conceptually* differ from the other types. To quote Guion (1977), '*All* validity is at its base some form of construct validity . . . . It *is* the basic meaning of validity' (p. 410).

It should not be surprising that given the greater complexity and breadth of questions asked with construct validity as compared with the other types of validity, there are many more ways of establishing it. In the next section, we will discuss only a few of these methods: extreme groups, convergent and discriminant validity, and the multitrait—multimethod matrix. Many other experimental and quasi-experimental approaches exist; the interested reader should consult some of the references listed in Appendix A.

Extreme groups
Perhaps the easiest experiment to conceive of in assessing the validity of a scale is to give it to two groups; one of which has the trait or behaviour, and the other which does not. The former group should score significantly higher (or lower, depending on how the items are scored) on the new instrument. This is sometimes called construct validation by *extreme groups*. We can use the attempt to develop a better scale for IBS as an example. Using their best tools, experienced clinicians would divide a group of patients presenting to a GI clinic into two sub-groups: those

whom they feel have IBS and those who have some other bowel disorder. To make the process of scale development easier, all patients with equivocal diagnoses would be eliminated in this type of study.

Although this type of design appears quite straightforward, it has buried within it two methodological problems. The first difficulty with the method is that if we are trying to develop a new or better tool, how can we select the extreme groups? To be able to do so would imply that there is already an instrument in existence which meets our needs. There is no ready solution to this problem. In practice, the groups are selected using the best *available* tool, even if it is the relatively crude criterion of 'expert judgement', or a scale that almost captures what our new scale is designed to tap. We can then use what Cronbach and Meehl (1955) call 'bootstrapping'. If the new scale allows us to make more accurate predictions, or explain more findings, or achieve better inter-observer agreement, then it can replace the original criterion. In turn, then, it can be used as the gold standard against which a newer or revised version can be validated; hence 'pulling ourselves up by the bootstraps'.

The second methodological problem is one that occurs with diagnostic tests, and which is often overlooked in the pressure to publish; the extreme group design may be a necessary step, but it is by no means sufficient. That is, it is minimally necessary for our new scale to be able to differentiate between those people who obviously have the disorder or trait in question and those who do not; if the scale cannot do this, it is probably useless in all other regards. However, the question must be asked, 'Is this the way the instrument will be used in practice?' If we are trying to develop a new diagnostic tool, the answer most often is 'no'. We likely would not need a new test to separate out the obvious cases from the obvious non-cases. Especially in a tertiary care setting, the people who are sent are in the middle range; they *may* have the disorder, but then again there are some doubts. If it is with this group that the instrument will be used, then the ultimate test of its usefulness is in making these much finer discriminations.

For example, many instruments have been designed to detect the presence of organic brain syndrome (OBS). As a first step, we would try out such a tool on one group of patients with confirmed brain damage and on another where there is no evidence of any pathology. These two groups should be clearly distinguishable on the new test. However, such patients are rarely referred for neuropsychological assessment, since their diagnoses (or lack thereof) are readily apparent based on other criteria. The next step, then, would be to try this instrument on the types of patients who *would* be sent for assessment, where the differential diagnosis is between OBS and depression, a difficult discrimination to make. These groups would be formed based on the best guess of a psychiatrist, perhaps augmented by some other tests of OBS, ones we are trying to replace.

Convergent and discriminant validity

Assessing the validity by using extreme groups is closely related to *convergent validity*; seeing how closely the new scale is related to other variables and other measures of the same construct to which it should be related. For example, if our theory states that anxious people are supposed to be more aware of autonomic nervous system (ANS) activity than non-anxious people, then scores on the new index of anxiety should correlate with scores on a measure of autonomic awareness. Again, if the scores do *not* correlate, then the problem can be our new scale, the measure of autonomic sensitivity, or our theory. On the other hand, we do not want the scales to be too highly correlated; this would indicate that they are measuring the same thing, that the new one is nothing more than a different measure of autonomic awareness. How high is 'too high?' As usual, it all depends. If ANS sensitivity is, by our theory, a major component of anxiety, then the correlation should be relatively robust; if it is only one of many components of anxiety, then the correlation should be lower.

The other aspect of convergent validity is that the new index of anxiety should correlate with other measures of this construct. Again, while the correlation should be high, it should not be overly high if we believe that our new anxiety scale covers components of this trait not tapped by the existing ones.

Not only should our construct correlate with related variables, it should *not* correlate with dissimilar, unrelated ones; what we refer to as *discriminant validity*. If our theory states that anxiety is independent of intelligence, then we should not find a strong correlation between the two. Finding one may indicate, for example, that the wording of our instrument is so difficult that intelligence is playing a role in simply understanding the items. Of course, the other reasons may also apply; our scale, the intelligence test, or the construct may be faulty.

The multitrait–multimethod matrix

A powerful technique for looking at convergent and discriminant validity simultaneously is called the *multitrait–multimethod* matrix, or MTMM (Campbell and Fiske 1959). Two or more different, usually unrelated, traits are each measured by two or more methods at the same time. The two traits, for instance, can be 'self-directed learning' and 'knowledge' (assuming that they are relatively unrelated), each assessed by a rater and a written exam. This leads to a matrix of 10 correlations, as shown with fictitious data in Table 10.2.

The numbers in parentheses (0.53, 0.79, etc.) along the main diagonal are the reliabilities of the four instruments. The two italicized figures, *0.42* and *0.49*, are the 'homotrait–heteromethod' correlations: the same trait (e.g. knowledge) measured in different ways. Those in curly brackets

Table 10.2 *A fictitious multitrait-multimethod matrix*

		Self-directed learning		Knowledge	
		Rater	Exam	Rater	Exam
Self-directed learning	Rater	(0.53)			
	Exam	0.42	(0.79)		
Knowledge	Rater	{0.18}	[0.17]	(0.58)	
	Exam	[0.15]	{0.23}	0.49	(0.88)

{0.18} and {0.23} are 'heterotrait–homomethod' correlations: different traits assessed by the same method. Finally, the heterotrait–heteromethod correlations are in square brackets [0.17] and [0.15]: different traits measured with different methods.

Ideally, the highest correlations should be the reliabilities of the individual measures; an examination of 'knowledge' given on two occasions should yield higher correlations than examinations of different traits or two different ways of tapping knowledge. Similarly, the lowest correlations should be the heterotrait—heteromethod ones; different traits measured by different methods should not be related.

Convergent validity is reflected in the homotrait–heteromethod correlations; different measures of the same trait should correlate with each other. In this example, the results of the written exam should correlate with scores given by the rater for 'knowledge', and similarly for the two assessments of 'self-directed learning'. Conversely, discriminant validity is shown by low correlations when the same method (e.g., the written exam) is applied to different traits—the heterotrait—homomethod coefficients. If they are as high or higher than the homotrait–heteromethod correlations, this would show that the *method* of measurement was more important than *what* was being measured. This is obviously an undesirable property, since the manner of assessing various attributes should be secondary to the relationship that should exist between various ways of tapping into the same trait.

It is often difficult to do studies appropriate for the MTMM approach because of the time required on the subjects' part, as well the problem of finding different methods of assessing the same trait. When these studies can be done, though, they can address a number of validity issues simultaneously.

Summary

Unlike criterion validity, then, there is no one experimental design or statistic which are common to construct validational studies. If one of the hypotheses is that our new measure of a construct is related to other indices of that construct or that the construct should be associated with other constructs, then the study is usually correlational in nature; our new scale and another one (of the same or a related construct) are given to the subjects. If one hypothesis is that some naturally occurring group has 'more' of the construct than another group, then we can simply give our new instrument to both groups, and look for differences between the two means. Still another hypothesis may be that if we give some experimental or therapeutic intervention, it will affect the construct and the measure of it; transcutaneous stimulation should reduce pain, while intense radiant heat should increase it. In this instance, our study could be a before–after trial or, more powerfully, a true experiment whereby one group receives the intervention and the other does not. If our construct is correct, and the manoeuvre worked, and our scale is valid, then we should see differences between the groups.

In summary, it is obviously necessary to conduct validational studies for each new instrument we develop. However, when the scale is one measuring a hypothetical construct, the task is an on-going one. New hypotheses derived from the construct require new studies. Similarly, if we want to use the measure with groups it was not initially validated on, we must first demonstrate that the inferences we make for them are as valid as for the original population. Finally, modifications of existing scales often require new validity studies. For example, if we wanted to use the D scale of the MMPI as an index of depression, we cannot assume that it is as valid when used in isolation as when the items are imbedded amongst 500 other, unrelated ones. It is possible that the mere fact of presenting them together gives the patient a different orientation and viewpoint.

Biases in validity assessment

Restriction in range

We mentioned in Chapter 8 that an unacceptable way of seeming to increase the reliability of a measure is to give it to a more heterogeneous group than the one it is designed for. In this section, we return to this point from a different perspective; how the range of scores affects the validity of the scale. There are actually three ways this can occur:
• the predictor variable (usually our new measure) is restricted;
• the criterion is restricted; and

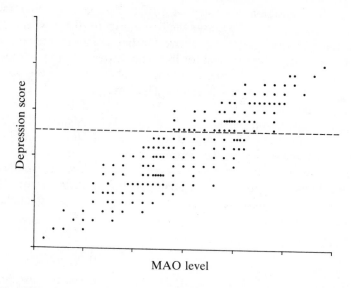

Fig. 10.1. Scatterplot showing the relationship between two variables.

- a third variable, correlated with both the predictor and criterion variables, is used to select the group which will be given the predictor and criterion variables.

As an example, assume that we have read about a new assay for serum monoamine oxidase (MAO) which is highly correlated with scores on a depression inventory. In the original (fictitious) article, a correlation of 0.80 was found in a large community-based sample. Such an assay would be extremely useful in a hospital setting, where difficulty with the English language and the various biases (e.g., faking good or bad) are often problems with self-administered scales. We replicate the study on our in-patient psychiatry ward, but find a disappointingly low correlation of only 0.37. Should we be surprised?

Based on our discussion of restriction of range, the answer is 'no'. We can illustrate this effect pictorially by drawing a scatter diagram of the two variables in the original study as in Figure 10.1.

As a brief reminder, a scatterplot is made by placing a dot at the intersection of a person's scores on the two variables. Alternatively, an ellipse can be drawn so that it includes (usually) 95 per cent of the people. The more elliptical the swarm of points or the ellipse, the stronger the correlation; the more circular the ellipse, the lower the association, with the extreme being a circle reflecting a total lack of any relationship. This scatterplot is fairly thin, as would be expected with a correlation of 0.80.

In our study, all of the subjects were hospitalized depressives, so their scores on the depression inventory are expected to be higher than those in a community sample, falling above the line in Figure 10.1. As can be seen, the portion of the ellipse falling above the line is more circular than the whole scatterplot, indicating that for this more restricted sample, the correlation between the two variables is considerably lower.

Using some equations developed by Thorndike (1949), we can predict how much the validity coefficient will be affected by selecting more restricted groups based on the criterion (X), the predictor (Y), or some other variable (Z). The first situation would apply if patients were hospitalized only if their scores on the depression inventory exceeded a certain level. This would be the case if high scores on the scale were one of the criteria for admission, and would be analogous to validating a new TB test only on patients who have lesions on an X-ray. In this case, the validity of the predictor would be:

$$r' = \frac{r\,(s'_x/s_x)}{\sqrt{[1 - r^2 + r^2\,(s'^2_x/s^2_x)]}}$$

where r' is the restricted validity coefficient, r is the validity coefficient in the unrestricted sample, s'_x is the SD of the criterion for the restricted sample, and s_x is the SD of the criterion for the unrestricted sample.

If the standard deviation in the unrestricted sample was 10, and it was reduced to 3 in the restricted sample, we would get:

$$\frac{0.80 \times (3/10)}{\sqrt{[1 - 0.64 + 0.64 \times (9/100)]}} = 0.37.$$

By the same token, we can work backwards by transforming this formula. If we did a study on a sample that was in some way constrained on the criterion variable, we could figure out what the validity coefficient would be if the full range of the variable were available. In this case, the formula would be:

$$r = \frac{r'\,(s_x/s'_x)}{\sqrt{[1 - r'^2 + r'^2\,(s^2_x/s'^2_x)]}}$$

where the terms have the same meaning as above.

The second case occurs when the group is selected on the basis of the *predictor* variable (Y); using the same example, only patients with increased MAO levels are included. This is the situation that obtains with criterion contamination; students are selected based on their scores on the admission test, which is actually being evaluated to see if it is a valid predictor. The formulae are the same, except that s'_y is substituted for s'_x, and s_y for s_x.

The last case is where the subjects are selected on the basis of some other variable (Z), which is correlated with both X and Y. Using our original example, this is the most realistic condition, since patients are admitted because of the severity of their symptomatology, which is related to both MAO level and scores on the depression inventory. The question can again be asked in two ways: (1) if we know the results from an (unrestricted) community-based study, what would the correlation be in our (more restricted) hospital environment; or (2), if we correlated X and Y in our restricted sample, what would the correlation be in an unrestricted one? Since an additional variable is involved (Z, the severity of depression), more information needs to be known: (1) the correlation of X and Y in the unrestricted sample; (2) the correlations of X with Z and Y with Z in this sample; and (3) the standard deviation of Z in the restricted and unrestricted samples. As these data are rarely known, the equation is mainly of academic interest. For those who are interested, a thorough treatment of this topic can be found in Ghiselli (1964).

Unreliability of the criterion

One pervasive problem in validation occurs when we correlate our new scale with a gold standard. Quite frequently, though, the criterion is not as good as this term suggests, since it is unreliable in its own right. Thus, the validity coefficient may be attenuated since, even if the predictor (Y) were excellent, it is predicting to an unreliable criterion (X). We can estimate what the validity coefficient would be if the criterion were perfectly reliable by using the formula:

$$r_{XY}' = \frac{r_{XY}}{\sqrt{(r_{XX})}}$$

where r_{XY}' is the estimated correlation with a perfectly reliable criterion, r_{XY} is the actual correlation between tests X and Y, and r_{XX} is the reliability coefficient of the criterion (test X).

If we assume that the criterion is perfectly reliable, and we want to see how much the correlation *could* improve if the new test were perfectly reliable, we would simply substitute r_{YY} for r_{XX} under the radical:

$$r_{XY}' = \frac{r_{XY}}{\sqrt{(r_{YY})}}.$$

A more general (and realistic) case assumes that both scales are unreliable, and we want to see what the correlation would be if both were perfectly reliable. The equation now reads:

$$r_{XY}' = \frac{r_{XY}}{\sqrt{(r_{XX}\,r_{YY})}}.$$

The most general (and realistic) case is that perfect reliability never exists, in either the new instrument or in the criterion. However, it may be possible to improve the reliability of one or both, and we would want to know what the correlation between the two indices would be, given these improved (albeit not perfect) reliabilities. In this case, we would use the equation:

$$r_{XY}' = \frac{r_{XY} \sqrt{(r_{XX}' \, r_{YY}')}}{\sqrt{(r_{XX} \, r_{YY})}}$$

where r_{XX}' and r_{YY}' are the changed reliabilities for the two variables (somewhere between their actual reliabilities and 1.0).

These equations have two possible uses. First, they tell us how much the validity would increase if we were able to increase the reliabilities of the instruments. If the increase is only marginal, then the investment of time and perhaps money needed to improve the psychometric properties may not be worth it; whereas a large potential increase may signal that it could be worthwhile making the investment. The second useful function is in the area of theory development. If our theory tells us that variable *A* should correlate strongly with variable *B*, then correcting for unreliability of the measures gives us an indication of the true validity of the instrument, and hence of our construct. A low, uncorrected validity estimate may incorrectly lead us to discard the theory, when in fact it may be correct, and the problem is with the scales.

By the same token, it is important to remember that these corrections for attenuation tells us what the validity *can be* if we could improve the reliability of the criterion and the new instrument, not what the validity *actually is* in real life. It is worth quoting Guion (1965) in this regard: 'The effect of a possible correction for attenuation should never be a consideration when one is deciding how to evaluate a measure as it exists' (p. 32).

Changes in the sample

Life would be simple if we could establish the validity of a measure once by conducting a series of studies, and then assume that we could use that instrument under a range of circumstances and with a variety of people. Unfortunately, this is not the case. Estimates of validity, like those of reliability, are dependent upon the nature of the people being measured and, to a greater or lesser degree, the circumstances under which they are being assessed. A tool which can accurately measure the activities of daily living among cancer patients may be quite useless when used in respirology; and one that has proven valid in distinguishing OBS from depressed patients may not discriminate between OBS patients and schizophrenics. Every time a scale is used in a new context, or with a different group of people, it is necessary to re-establish its psychometric properties.

Summary

Validity is a process of determining what, if anything, we are measuring with our scale; that is, can we make valid statements about a person based on his or her score on the index. *Concurrent* validity is most often used when we are trying to replace one tool with a simpler, cheaper, or less invasive one. We generally use another form of criterion validation, called *predictive* validity, in developing instruments that allow us to get answers earlier than current instruments allow. *Construct validity* refers to a wide range of approaches which are used when what we are trying to measure is a 'hypothetical construct,' like anxiety or some syndromes, rather than something which can be readily observed.

References

Campbell, D. T., and Fiske, D. W. (1959). Convergent and discriminant validation by the multitrait-multimethod matrix. *Psychological Bulletin*, **56**, 81–105.

Cattell, R. B. (1963). Theory of fluid and crystallized intelligence: Critical experiment. *British Journal of Educational Psychology*, **54**, 1–22.

Cronbach, L. J. (1971). Test validation. In *Educational measurement* (ed. R. L. Thorndike), pp. 221–37. American Council on Education, Washington DC.

Cronbach, L. J., and Meehl, P. E. (1955) Construct validity in psychological tests. *Psychological Bulletin*, **52**, 281–302.

Ghiselli, E. E. (1964). *Theory of psychological measurement*. McGraw-Hill, New York.

Guion, R. M. (1965). *Personnel testing*. McGraw-Hill, New York.

Guion, R. M. (1977). Content validity: Three years of talk—what's the action? *Public Personnel Management*, **6**, 407–14.

Landy, F. J. (1986). Stamp collecting versus science. *American Psychologist*, **41**, 1183–92.

Messick, S. (1980). Test validity and the ethics of assessment. *American Psychologist*, **35**, 1012–27.

Thorndike, R. L. (1949). *Personnel selection: Test and measurement techniques*. Wiley, New York.

11

Measuring change

Introduction

The measurement of change has been a topic of considerable confusion in the medical literature. As clinicians and researchers, we view that the ultimate goal of most treatment—medical, surgical, psychosocial, or educational—is to induce change in the patient's or student's status. It would appear to follow that the measurement of change in patients' health state or in a student's level of understanding is an appropriate goal of research. A number of recent articles (Guyatt *et al.* 1987; MacKenzie *et al.* 1986) have advocated this position, both on the grounds that the measurement of change in patient's condition is the goal of clinical care and should be addressed by research methods, and on the methodological basis that instruments which are responsive to changes in health status are more sensitive measures of the effects of clinical interventions than those which simply assess health status after an intervention.

However, this opinion is by no means unanimous. Several authors in education and psychology have taken stands against the use of difference scores (Cronbach and Furby 1970; Burckhardt *et al.* 1982). In this chapter, we explore the issues surrounding the use of change scores and show that these divergent positions are based on different views of the goals of measurement, and different assumptions regarding the methodological advantages and disadvantages of change measures.

The goal of measurement of change

In order to understand the source of the controversy in the literature, it is necessary to recognize that the measurement of change can be directed at different goals. These have been described by Linn and Slinde (1977).

1. *To measure differences between individuals in the amount of change.* Although apparently similar to the notion of reliability, the intent is to dis-

tinguish between those individuals who *change a lot* and those who *change little*. For example, if we wanted to identify individuals who were responsive to therapy (e.g. in a secondary analysis of a trial of therapy for arthritis), we would proceed by a comparison of individual differences in change scores. Much of the literature in psychology addressing the measurement of change accepts this as the basic goal of change measurement.

2. *To identify correlates of change.* This goal really represents an elaboration of the first. If we were successful at identifying responsive sub-groups in a trial of therapy, a logical second step is to attempt to identify those factors which are associated or correlated with good response. The issues of measurement also follow from the earlier concerns: if we cannot differentiate between those who change a great deal and those who change little, the resulting restriction in range will attenuate any attempt to find correlates.

3. *To infer treatment effects from group differences.* This goal is probably the primary goal of most clinical trials. By randomly assigning individuals to treatment and control groups, measuring the health state before and after treatment, and then comparing the average change in health state in the groups, we can determine a treatment effect—individuals in a treatment group will change, on the average, more than those in a control group.

The first and last goals work against one another. To the extent that there are individual differences in response to treatment, this is an indication that the treatment had different effects on different people, and it will be more difficult to detect an overall treatment effect. However, if there are individual differences in response to treatment, then we will be able to identify responsive sub-groups and possible prognostic factors; if there are no individual differences, we will be unsuccessful in this search.

Note however, that there is no conflict in the goal of discrimination between individuals, as expressed in the reliability coefficient, and the goal of evaluation of change within individuals. It is certainly possible that there may be large and stable differences between individuals on some measure, yet all may change equally in response to treatment. If we consider the everyday example of dieting, overweight people may range from 60 kg to 150 kg; yet a conservative and successful diet would have all losing from 1 to 2 kg per week. As long as there was reasonable consistency in the amount of weight loss experienced by different individuals in the plan, it would not be difficult to demonstrate the efficacy of a treatment program which showed losses of this order, despite the large differences in individual weights. So the presence of large differences among individuals does not, of itself, preclude the demonstration of small treatment effects. Differences in *change* of different individuals *does* reduce the chance of demonstrating overall treatment effects.

Table 11.1 *Weight (in kg) of six patients in a diet clinic*

Patient	Before	After two weeks	Average	Change
1	150	144	147	−6
2	120	112	116	−8
3	110	108	109	−2
4	140	142	141	+2
5	138	132	135	−6
6	116	112	114	−4
Mean	129	125	127	−4.0

Measures of association—reliability, and sensitivity to change

The different goals of measurement are reflected in different coefficients, analogous to the reliability coefficient, which express the ability of an instrument to detect change within subjects or the effects of treatment. In order to clarify these distinctions, let us consider a group of six individuals who have entered into a diet plan and are weighed before treatment and again after two weeks of dieting. The data, might look like Table 11.1 above.

As we discussed before, the goal of discriminating among subjects has been incorporated in the notion of *reliability*, which we discussed at length in Chapter 8, and is defined as:

$$\text{Reliability } (R) = \frac{\sigma^2_{\text{pat}}}{\sigma^2_{\text{pat}} + \sigma^2_{\text{err}}}.$$

In the present example, the reliability focuses on the difference between patients' average weights, and σ^2_{pat} would be determined from a sum of squares calculated as:

$$SS_{\text{pat}} = (147-127)^2 + (116-127)^2 + \ldots + (147-127)^2.$$

By analogy, we can also develop a measure to describe the reproducibility of the change score, i.e. an index of the ability of the measure to discriminate between those subjects who change a great deal and those who change little.

Reliability of the change score

The assessment of the ability of an instrument to detect individual differences in change scores is appropriately labelled as the *reliability of the change score* (Lord and Novick, 1968). By analogy to the reliability coefficient, this can be expressed as:

$$\text{Reliability } (D) = \frac{\sigma^2_D}{\sigma^2_D + \sigma^2_{err}(D)}$$

where σ^2_D expresses the systematic difference between subjects in their change score, and $\sigma^2_{err}(D)$ is the error associated with this estimate. In our example, σ^2_D would be derived from a sum of squares calculated as:

$$SS_D = (-6-(-4))^2 + (-8-(-4))^2 + \ldots + (-4-)-4))^2.$$

The reliability of the change score can be shown to be related to the variance of pre-test (x) and post-test (y) scores, their reliability (R) and the correlation between pre-test and post-test (r), in the following manner:

$$\text{Reliability } (D) = \frac{\sigma_x^2 R_{xx} + \sigma_y^2 R_{yy} - 2\sigma_x\sigma_y r_{xy}}{\sigma_x^2 + \sigma_y^2 - 2\sigma_x\sigma_y r_{xy}}$$

where r_{xy} is the correlation between the pre-test and post-test. If the pre-test and post-test have the same variances, this expression reduces to:

$$\text{Reliability} = \frac{R_{xx} + R_{yy} - 2r_{xy}}{2.0 - 2r_{xy}}$$

where R_x and R_y are the reliabilities of the initial and final measurements. In our previous example, the measured reliability was 0.95. If we assume that this reliability coefficient applies equally to both pre-test and post-test, and we further assume a correlation of, e.g. 0.80 between the two measures, then the reliability of the difference score becomes:

$$\text{Reliability } (D) = \frac{0.95 + 0.95 - 2 \times 0.80}{2.0 - 2 \times 0.80} = 0.30/0.40 = 0.75.$$

In the limiting case, it can be demonstrated that, under the circumstances where there is a perfect correlation between the pre-test and post-test scores, the reliability of the difference score is zero. Although this appears strange, it actually follows from the basic notion of discriminating between those who change a great deal and those who change little. If an experimental intervention resulted in a uniform response to treatment, all patients would improve an equal amount. As a result, the variance of the change score will be zero, since every patient's post-test score would be equal to his or her pre-test score except for a constant; no patients would have changed more or less than any other, and the reliability of the difference score would be zero.

Since a perfectly uniform response to treatment would represent an ideal state of affairs for the use of change scores to measure treatment effects, yet would yield a reliability coefficient for change scores of zero, it should not be used as an index appropriate for assessing the ability of an instrument to measure treatment effects, and some other approach must be used.

Sensitivity to change resulting from treatment effects

The preceding discussion suggests that it would be useful to devise some measure analogous to the reliability coefficient to describe an instrument's ability to detect the overall effect of treatments. This effect has been variously labelled as 'sensitivity to change' and 'responsiveness' in the literature. In contrast to the assessment of individual differences in change, there is no consensus regarding the appropriate measure of the sensitivity of a measure to the main effect of treatment. Some approaches use the magnitude of the statistical test (e.g. an F-ratio) to estimate sensitivity to treatment effects; other methods use various measures of the strength of effect, expressed as a ratio of the difference between groups to the variability within groups.

One approach builds on the assumptions of generalizability theory, discussed in the previous chapter. We can conceptualize the effect of treatment as a 'facet of differentiation', i.e. a variance component of interest, and all other interactions as 'facets of generalization' over which we want to estimate the effect of treatment. Then we can proceed to construct a generalizability coefficient as a ratio of variances.

Returning to the example of Table 11.1, the variance component of interest in examining treatment effects is related to the average difference between post-treatment and pre-treatment scores, so is derived from a sum of squares* like

$$SS_{tr} = (125 - 129)^2.$$

In fact, it would be usual to attempt to evaluate treatment effects from pre-post differences in the absence of a control group, as any observed differences could be due to other explanations than the effect of treatment. More commonly, a control group would be included, and measures taken before and after treatment on both treatment and control groups. An example could be a second evaluation of diet, obtained by randomizing ten patients to treatment and control groups, then weighing each patient before and after a period of treatment. The data might resemble Table 11.2.

The appropriate statistical analysis would be to compare the difference scores of the treatment group to those of the control group using an

---

* Although the sums of squares we have calculated are useful for understanding the conceptual differences among the three measures of association, the actual sum of squares would be obtained by multiplying these calculated squared differences by the appropriate n's.

Table 11.2 *Hypothetical data from patients at a weight loss clinic*

	Subject	Pre-test	Post-test	Difference
	1	80	72	−8
	2	75	71	−4
Diet	3	70	63	−7
	4	65	55	−10
	5	60	54	−6
Mean		70.0	63.0	−7.0
Standard deviation			8.51	2.23
	6	80	81	+1
	7	75	72	−3
Control	8	70	73	+3
	9	65	64	−1
	10	60	60	0
Mean		70.0	70.0	0.0
Standard deviation			8.21	2.23

unpaired *t*-test on the difference scores, or to conduct a repeated measures analysis of variance, which is mathematically equivalent, and examine the interaction between time and treatment.

The results of the analysis are shown in the ANOVA table in Table 11.3. The test of significance of the time x treatment interaction involves the ratio of the mean square of the interaction, 61.25, and the mean square error, 2.50; it is expressed as an *F*-ratio:

$$F(1,8) = 61.25/2.50 = 24.50.$$

Table 11.3 *Analysis of variance of diet clinic data*

Source	Sum of squares	d.f.	Mean square
Between subjects			
Treatments	61.25	1	61.25
Subjects	1040.0	8	130.00
Within subjects			
Pre-post	61.25	1	61.25
Pre-post treat	61.25	1	61.25
Residual error	200.0	8	2.50

This ratio is exactly the square of an equivalent t-test, examining the mean difference score in the two groups.

Regardless of the statistical test employed (t-test of difference scores or ANOVA) in the present example, analysis of difference scores comparing treatment and control groups is the method of choice because it removes the effect of stable differences between individuals and results in a more powerful statistical test.

We can now return to the original purpose of developing a measure of sensitivity to change. As we indicated, the effect of the weight loss plan was contained in the pre-post x treatment interaction, whose variance can be estimated using the methods described in Chapters 8 and 9. In this example, the expected mean square (EMS) is equal to

$$\text{EMS} = \sigma^2_{err} + 5\sigma^2_{interaction}.$$

Working through this equation yields an estimated variance of 11.75. The error in this estimate was contributed by the subjects x pre-post interaction, equal to 2.50. These values can then be incorporated into a sensitivity to change coefficient, equal to

$$\text{Sensitivity} = \frac{\sigma^2_{change}}{\sigma^2_{change} + \sigma^2_{err}}$$

$$= \frac{11.75}{11.75 + 2.50} = 0.825.$$

The resulting coefficient expresses the proportion of the variance in the change score due to 'true', i.e. experimentally induced change. As such, it ranges from 0 to 1, and is on the same metric as the reliability coefficient. Note that the reliability coefficient and sensitivity coefficient are related but not identical. Both use the same error term, but their magnitude is related to the relative magnitude of the pre–post variance and the variance due to patients.

Difficulties with change scores in experimental designs

Potential loss of precision

Although it would appear that it is always desirable to measure change since it removes the effect of variance between patients, this is actually not the case. The calculation of a difference score is based on the difference between two quantities, the pre-test and post-test, and both are measured with some error, σ^2_{err}. If this quantity is sufficiently large relative to the variance between patients, the net result might be to introduce more, rather than less, error into the estimate of treatment effect.

The conditions under which it makes sense to measures change within patients as measure of treatment effect can be expressed in terms of a generalizability coefficient. The use of change scores to estimate treatment main effects is only appropriate when the variance between subjects exceeds the error variance within subjects. This is equivalent to the following expression:

$$\frac{\sigma^2_{sub}}{\sigma^2_{sub} + \sigma^2_{err}} \geq 0.5.$$

Thus, one should only use change scores when the reliability of the measure exceeds 0.5. Reliability is not irrelevant or inversely related to sensitivity—*reliability is a necessary pre-condition for the appropriate application of change scores.* This analysis does not, of course, imply that measures which are reliable are, of necessity, useful for the assessment of change. Even if an instrument is reliable, it remains to be shown that differences in response to treatment can be detected before the instrument can be used for the assessment of change.

Biased measurement of treatment effects

The simple subtraction of post-treatment from pre-treatment scores to create a difference score as a measure of the overall effect of treatment assumes that the effect of treatment will be the same, except for random error, for all patients. This assumption can be shown to be false in many, if not most circumstances. One reason is that one major cause of an individual having an extreme score on pretest is simply an accumulation of random processes; i.e. the very good scores are to some extent due to good luck, and the very bad scores are due to bad luck. To the extent that chance is operative (and any reliability coefficient less than 1 is an indication of the presence of random variation), then the very good are likely to get worse, and the very bad get better, on retest. This effect is known as 'regression to the mean'. In effect, the best line fitting post-test to pre-treatment data in the absence of treatment effects has a slope less than 1 and an intercept greater than 0. The use of change scores assumes a best fit line with a slope of 1 and intercept of 0. The consequence of regression to the mean is that the use of change or difference scores overestimates the effect of pre-test differences on post-test scores.

The solution to this problem for assessing individual change recommended by Cronbach and Furby (1970) is the use of *residualized gain scores.* Instead of subtracting pre-test from post-test, we first fit the line relating the pre-test and post-test scores using regression analysis. We then estimate the post-test score of each patient from the regression equation. The residualized gain score is the difference between the actual post-test score and the score which was predicted from the regression equation. In other words, the residualized gain score removes from consideration that portion of the gain score which was linearly predictable from the pre-test score. What remains is an indication of those individuals who changed more or less than was expected.

This operation is really designed to identify individual differences in change in an unbiased manner. Cronbach and Furby (1970) among others have commented on the use of change scores to estimate overall treatment effects, and conclude that analysis of covariance methods should be employed when the reliability is sufficiently large, and simple post-test scores otherwise.

The reason for the use of ANCOVA is again related to the phenomenon of regression to the mean. As we discussed, the change score assumes that the line relating pre-test to post-test has a slope of 1 and intercept 0, which is not the optimal line when error of measurement is present. The result is that the denominator of the statistical test of treatment effects includes variance due to lack of fit, resulting in a conservate test. Since ANCOVA fits an optimum line to the data, in general, this will result in a smaller error term and a more sensitive test of treatment effects.

Change scores and quasi-experimental designs

So far, we have addressed the use of change scores in the context of randomized trials, where the primary goal is to increase the sensitivity of statistical tests by reducing the magnitude of the error term. There is another potential application of these methods in situations such as cohort analytical studies where there are likely to be initial differences between treatment and control groups. In this situation, the change score has an apparent advantage, in that the subtraction of the initial score for each subject will have the effect of eliminating the initial differences between groups.

However, when the change score is used in a situation where there are differences between the two groups on the pre-test measure, as might result if subjects were not allocated at random to the two conditions, additional complications arise. These are directly related to the effect of regression to the mean, discussed in the section on residualized gain scores. In the absence of treatment effects, individuals measured with some random error will not stay the same on retest. Those who were very good will worsen, on average, and those who were very bad will improve.

Unfortunately this effect also applies to group means, which are simply the average of individual scores. In the absence of any treatment effect, the differences between groups will be reduced at the second testing, con-

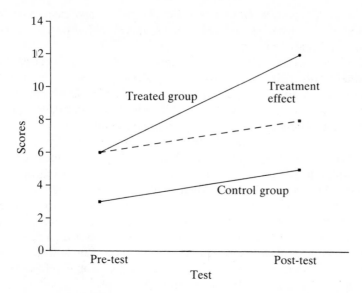

Fig. 11.1. Relation between pre-test and post-test scores in a quasi-experimental design

founding any interpretation of differences between groups observed following treatment. One way around this problem is again the use of *analysis of covariance*, however this method is a refinement to the use of change scores, not a fundamentally different approach.

There are other fundamental reasons to view any attempt at post-hoc adjustment for differences between groups on pretest, whether by difference scores, repeated measures ANOVA or ANCOVA, with considerable suspicion. Implicit in these analytical methods is a specific model of the change process which cannot be assumed to have general applicability. This is illustrated in Figure 11.1.

Any of the analytical methods assume that, in the absence of any treatment effect, the experimental and control group will grow at the same rate, so that the difference in means at the beginning would equal the difference in means at the end, and any additional difference between the two groups (shown as the difference between the post-test mean of the treated group and the dotted line) is evidence of a treatment effect.

Unfortunately, there are any number of plausible alternative models which will fit the data equally well. For example, in a rehabilitation setting or in an educational program for mentally handicapped children, individuals who are less impaired, thus score higher initially, may have the greatest capacity for change or improvement over time. Under these circumstances, referred to in the literature as a 'fan-spread' model, the observed data would be obtained in the absence of any treatment effect, and ANCOVA or analysis of difference scores would wrongly conclude a benefit from treatment.

Conversely, a situation may arise where a 'ceiling effect' occurs; that is, individuals with high scores initially may already be at the limit of their potential, thus would be expected to improve relatively less with treatment than those with initially lower scores. In this circumstance, the post-test scores in the absence of an effect of treatment would converge, and the analysis would underestimate the treatment effect.

It is evident that any analysis based on just one or two means for each group will not permit a choice among these models of growth, and additional points on the individual growth curve would be required (Rogosa *et al.* 1982). Of course, if such situations were rare, one could argue for the adequacy of change score approaches; however it is likely that situations of non-constant growth are the rule, not the exception, in health research. As Lord (1967) put it, 'there simply is no logical or statistical procedure that can be counted on to make proper allowances for uncontrolled preexisting differences between groups'.

Summary

This chapter has attempted to resolve some controversies surrounding the measurement of change. There are two distinct purposes for measuring change—examining overall effects of treatments and distinguishing individual differences in treatment response. Focusing on the former, we demonstrated that reliability and sensitivity to change are different but related concepts. We determined the conditions under which the measurement of change will result in increased and decreased statistical power. We also reviewed the literature on the use of change scores to correct for baseline differences and concluded that this purpose can rarely be justified.

References

Burckhardt, C.S., Goodwin, L.D., and Prescott, P.A. (1982). The measurement of change in nursing schools: Statistical considerations. *Nursing Research*, **31**, 53–5.
Cronbach, L.J. and Furby, L. (1970). How should we measure 'change'—or should we? *Psychological Bulletin*, **74**, 68–80.
Guyatt, G., Walter, S.D., and Norman, G.R. (1987). Measuring change over time: Assessing the usefulness of evaluative instruments. *Journal of Chronic Diseases*, **40**, 171–8.
Linn, P.L. and Slinde, J.A. (1977). Determination of the significance of change between pre- and posttesting periods. *Reviews of Educational Research*, **47**, 121–50.

Lord, F.M. (1967). A paradox in the interpretation of group comparisons. *Psychological Bulletin*, **68**, 304–5.

Lord, F.M. and Novick, M.N. (1968). *Statistical theories of mental test development*. Addison-Wesley, Reading, MA.

MacKenzie, C.R., Charlson, M.E., DiGioia, D., and Kelley, K. (1986). Can the Sickness Impact Profile measure change: An example of scale assessment. *Journal of Chronic Diseases*, **39**, 429–38.

Rogosa, D., Brandt, D., and Zimowski, M. (1982). A growth curve approach to the measurement of change. *Psychological Bulletin*, **92**, 726–48.

Latent-trait theory

Another approach to test construction is based on *latent-trait* (or *item response*) *theory*. This theory states that a person's performance on a specific test item is determined by the amount of the underlying trait (usually referred to by the Greek letter, θ, theta) that the person has; where he or she falls on the continuum of the trait. 'Performance' on an achievement type of test means answering the question correctly; on an attitudinal test, it refers to responding in the direction reflecting more of that trait. The assumption (which is testable, although often untested) is that the test is unidimensional, in that it taps only the one underlying trait and nothing else. A 'latent trait' does not refer to some underlying psychological construct; it is, rather, a statistical concept to explain the consistency of people's responses to the items in the scale.

Item characteristic curves

Figure 12.1 depicts hypothetical curves showing the response to two questions, A and B, on a test of some trait. These are called *item characteristic curves* (ICCs). A few important characteristics of the curves are worth noting. They are similar to one another in two ways. First, they are both S shaped (the technical name for the shape is an 'ogive'). While other shapes of the ICC are possible, the ogive is the most widely used one in test construction. Second, they are *monotonic*; the probability of answering in a positive direction consistently increases as the score on the latent trait increases. However, they differ from each other along three dimensions: the steepness of their slopes; their location along the trait continuum; and where they flatten out on the bottom. We shall return to the significance of these differences shortly.

For illustrative purposes, we have drawn a horizontal line where the probability is 0.5; it intersects Question A at value of the trait of 10, and Question B at a value of 14. Strictly speaking, a '50 per cent probability' does *not* mean that a given individual has a 50 per cent chance of responding to the question positively; rather, it means that if we took 100 people with the same amount of the trait, 50 of them will answer one way and 50

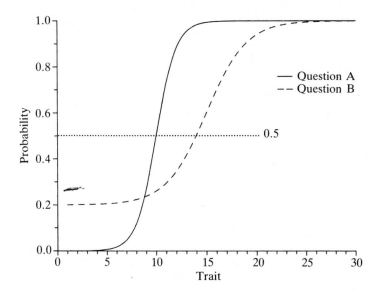

Fig. 12.1. Hypothetical item characteristic curves for two items.

the other way. (Models have been developed to handle items with more than two responses, but they are computationally quite difficult, and few computer programs exist to handle these cases.)

What can we tell from these two curves? First, Question A is probably a better discriminator of the trait than Question B. The reason is that the proportion of people responding in the positive direction changes relatively rapidly on Question A as the value of the trait increases. The slope for Question B is flatter, indicating that it does not discriminate as well. For example, as we move from a trait value of 5 to 15, the proportion of people answering positively to Question A increases from 1 per cent to 99 per cent; while for Question B, a comparable 10-point change in the trait is associated with an increase only from 26 per cent to 94 per cent. When the curve has the maximum steepness, it takes the form of a 'step function'; no people below the critical point respond positively, and everyone above it responds in the positive direction. The items would then form a perfect Guttman type of scale. Thus, one way of thinking about item response curves is that they are 'imperfect' Guttman scales, where the probability of responding increases gradually with more of the trait, rather than jumping from a probability of 0 to 100 per cent.

A second observation is that Question B is 'harder' than Question A throughout most of the range of the trait. That is, the average person needs more of the trait in order to respond in the positive direction. This can be

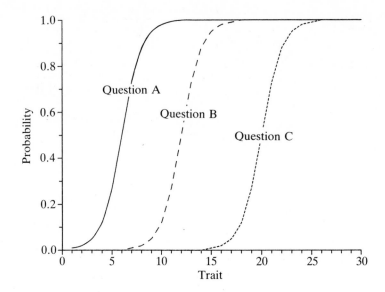

Fig. 12.2. Item characteristic curves for three items with equal discrimination but different levels of difficulty.

seen by the fact that the 50 per cent point is further along the trait continuum for Question B than it is for Question A.

Different models

When latent-trait theory was first developed, a simplifying assumption was made that the ICC ogives were all based on a normal distribution of scores. This assumption has been replaced by three 'models' which are likely more accurate descriptions of the distribution of responses. The simplest is the *one-parameter model*, which is also referred to as the *Rasch model* (Rasch 1960; Wright 1977). According to this model, the only factor affecting the ICCs of the various items in a test is the item difficulty, denoted b_i. That is, it assumes that all of the items have equal discriminating ability (designated as a). This is reflected in that the slopes of all the curves are parallel, but they are placed at various points along the trait continuum, as in Figure 12.2.

Formally, the proportion of people who have θ amount of the trait who answer item i correctly is given as:

$$P_i(\theta) = \frac{\exp\{a(\theta - b_i)\}}{1 + \exp\{a(\theta - b_i)\}}.$$

Since the form of this equation is called 'logistic', this and the other two models are referred to as *logistic models* or *logistic ogive models*.

The *two-parameter model* holds that the ICCs differ from each other on the basis of both difficulty and discriminating ability; that is, instead of *a* being a constant, there is a different a_i for each item. Now the ICCs differ from each other in two ways; the position along the trait line, and the slope of the curve, as seen in Figure 12.3.

The equation for this takes the form

$$P_i(\theta) = \frac{\exp\{a_i(\theta - b_i)\}}{1 + \exp\{a_i(\theta - b_i)\}} .$$

Both of these models assume that at the lowest level of the trait, the probability of responding positively is zero; that is, the left tail of all of the curves is asymptotic to the *x*-axis. This may be a valid assumption if the test is a personality or attitudinal questionnaire. However, with achievement tests, such as multiple-choice questionnaires, it is likely that people will guess on questions to which they do not know the answer, and get a certain proportion of those items correct by chance. The *three-parameter model* takes this into account, and allows the lower end of the curve to asymptote

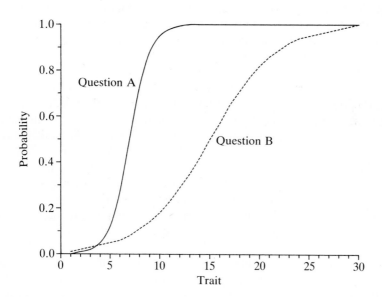

Fig. 12.3. Item characteristic curves for two items differing in both discrimination and difficulty.

at some probability level greater than 0. This 'pseudo-guessing parameter' is designated as c_i, and the resulting equation is given as:

$$P_i(\theta) = c_i + \frac{(1 - c_i) \exp \{a_i(\theta - b_i)\}}{1 + \exp \{a_i(\theta - b_i)\}} .$$

An example of a curve where c_i is 0.2 rather than 0.0 is Question B in Figure 12.1.

Deriving the curves

The mechanics of deriving ICCs involve taking a large number of subjects (a minimum of 200 for estimating a one-parameter model, and some authors have recommended using as many as 1000 to estimate the three parameters accurately), for whom we know or can estimate their value of the trait. If we do not have enough information to estimate the trait, then we must make some assumptions about its distribution, and sample people who span the range of the trait. The first step is to calculate the proportion of people at each level of the trait who answer each question in the positive direction. Most computer programs, such as BICAL (Wright *et al.* 1980), which is based on the one-parameter model, or LOGIST (Wingersky 1983), which can estimate the three-parameter one, then determine if the items meet the underlying assumption of unidimensionality. This is most often done by factor analysing the item correlation matrix; unidimensionality would be reflected in a large, dominant first factor, with the remaining factors being relatively weak.

The next step is to decide whether to use a one-, two-, or three-parameter model. While this decision *should* be based on the underlying theory one has about the trait and empirical comparisons of the results, it is more often determined by pragmatic issues: far larger samples are needed to estimate the slope and guessing parameters, and most of the available computer programs are based on the one-parameter Rasch model. With the data for the proportion of people responding positively to each item and the model to be used, the program then can compute the necessary parameters for each item. The specific mathematics of calculating ICCs are beyond the scope of this book, and require a computer if the results are needed in a reasonable time. Those who want to delve deeper into this topic should see Lord (1980).

The latent-trait model differs from the more traditional, random sampling, approach to test construction in a number of ways. With the latter, the items are assumed to be randomly chosen from a universe of possible items, and the person's score is the number of items responded to positively. Each item can thus be seen as, in some sense, equivalent to each other item. The latent-trait model, on the other hand, postulates a known relationship between the response to a specific item and the underlying trait; each item stands alone, having a different difficulty parameter. One trade-off is that for the random sampling approach, it is necessary to start with a large pool of items, but it is not necessary to know much about the items before item selection begins. Far fewer items are needed with the latent-trait approach, but more needs to be known about the item–trait relationship.

Advantages and disadvantages

The major potential advantage of ICC scaling is that it allows *test-free measurement*; that is, people can be compared to one another on the trait even if they took different items! Assume that we have developed a test of physical mobility, using latent-trait theory, and have come up with 30 items which span the range from complete immobility at the low end to unrestricted mobility at the top. These items can be thought of as comprising a Guttman-ordered scale; responding positively to the eighth item, for example, means that the person must have responded positively to the previous seven items. Conversely, if a person answers in the negative direction to item 15, then he or she would not answer positively to any item above number 15. Knowing this, we need not give all of the items to all people, only those items which span the point where the person switches from answering in one direction to answering in the other. That point places the person at a specific point on the mobility continuum. Since an underlying assumption of latent-trait theory is that the test is unidimensional, the point can be directly compared to that of another person, who was given a different subset of the items. In actuality, since the slopes are not vertical as with a Guttman scale, a number of items spanning the critical point must be used.

This form of scaling has received its widest application in achievement testing. Many of the newer tests, such as the revised version of the *Wide Range Achievement Test* (Jastak and Wilkinson 1984), the *Keymath Diagnostic Arithmetic Test* (Connolly *et al.* 1976), and the *Woodcock Reading Mastery Tests* (Woodcock 1973) have used it, so that people at different levels can be given different items, yet be placed on the same scale at the end. This means that people with less of the trait (e.g. spelling ability) are not frustrated by being given a large number of items which are beyond their ability; nor are people with more of the trait bored by having to spell very easy words like 'cat' or 'run'. In addition to reducing frustration, it also reduces testing time, since candidates do not spend large amounts of time on items which are trivial or beyond their ability. This 'adaptive' or 'tailored' testing is not dependent on item response theory, but is greatly facilitated by it.

Despite these advantages, latent-trait theory has not been widely used in test construction. One primary reason is the relatively large sample size needed to accurately estimate the item parameters. While groups of 1000 may be feasible in developing a test that will be used commercially or used for national certification examinations, it is usually infeasible for research purposes or local applications. A second reason is that, in many situations, the assumptions of the one-parameter Rasch model are difficult to meet. In order to find items with equivalent discrimination parameters and which asymptotically approach 0, a large number of items must be initially tested, obviating one potential advantage of the technique. Third, one of the mathematical assumptions of latent-trait theory is 'local independence'. This holds that, for any given level of the trait, the probabilities $P_i(\theta)$ are independent. This then rules out using questions which are chained (the answer to one is dependent upon the answer to previous items), or where the context created by previous questions affects the response to later items. Last, and perhaps most important, latent-trait theory assumes that the item parameters are the same across samples, especially when these samples are drawn from populations situated at different points along the trait continuum. If the items are tested in a number of different groups, then as Choppin (1976) states, 'eventually every item will show discrepancies; every item can be discarded; no item fits the model exactly' (p. 238).

References

Choppin, B. H. (1976). Recent developments in item banking. In *Advances in psychological and educational measurement* (eds. D. N. M. De Gruitjer and L. J. van der Kamp), pp. 233–45. Wiley, New York.

Connolly, A. J., Nachtman, W., and Pritchett, E. M. (1976). *Keymath Diagnostic Arithmetic Test*. American Guidance Service, Circle Pines MN.

Jastak, S. and Wilkinson, G. S. (1984). *The Wide Range Achievement Test - Revised: Administration manual*. Jastak Associates, Wilmington.

Lord, F. M. (1980). *Application of item response theory to practical testing problems*. Erlbaum, Hillsdale NJ.

Rasch, G. (1960). *Probabilistic models for some intelligence and attainment tests*. Nielson and Lydiche, Copenhagen.

Wingersky, M. S. (1983). LOGIST: A program for computing maximum likelihood procedures for logistic test models. In *Applications of item response theory* (ed. R. K. Hambleton), pp. 45–56. Educational Research Institute of British Columbia, Vancouver.

Woodcock, R. W. (1973). *Woodcock Reading Mastery Tests manual*. American Guidance Service, Circle Pines MN:

Wright, B. D. (1977). Solving measurement problems with the Rasch model. *Journal of Educational Measurement*, **14**, 97–116.

Wright, B. D., Mead, R. J., and Bell, S. R. (1980). *BICAL: Calibrating items with the Rasch model* (Research Memorandum No. 23C). University of Chicago, Department of Education Statistical Laboratory.

13

Methods of administration

Having developed the questionnaire, the next problem is how to administer it. This is an issue which not only affects costs and response rates, but, as we shall see, may influence which questions can be asked and in what format. The three methods commonly used to administer questionnaires are face-to-face interviews, over the telephone, and by mail.

As the cost of microcomputers has come down, scales can now be 'administered' by a computer, with the respondent sitting in front of a terminal. At the present time, this is possible primarily within clinical contexts where the subject is already near the researcher's office, or as part of smaller studies. However, as 'lap top' computers become more powerful, computer presentation will become more prevalent. Each of these methods has its own distinct advantages and disadvantages, which will be discussed in this chapter.

Face-to-face interviews

As the name implies, this method involves a trained interviewer administering the scale or questionnaire on a one-to-one basis, either in an office or, more usually, in the subject's home. The latter setting serves to put the respondents at ease, since they are in familiar surroundings, and may also increase compliance, because the subjects do not have to travel. However, home interviewing involves greater cost to the investigator and the possibility of interruptions, for instance, by telephones or family members.

Advantages

The advantages of face-to-face interviewing begin even before the first question is asked—the interviewer is sure who is responding. This is not the case with telephone or mail administration, since anyone in the household can answer or provide a second opinion for the respondent. In addition, having to respond verbally to another person reduces the number of items omitted by the respondent; it is more difficult to refuse to answer than simply to omit an item on a form (Quine 1985). The interviewer can also determine if the subject is having any difficulty understanding the items, whether due to a poor grasp of the language, limited intelligence, problems in concentration, or boredom. Further, since many immigrants and people with limited education understand the spoken language better than they can read it, and read it better than they can write it, fewer people will be eliminated because of these problems. This method of administration also allows the interviewer to rephrase the question in terms the person may better understand, or to probe for a more complete response. The converse of this, though, is that without sufficient training, the interviewer may distort the meaning of questions.

Another advantage is the flexibility afforded in presenting the items, since questions in an interview can range from 'closed' to 'open'. Closed questions, which require only a number as a response, such as the person's age, number of children, or years of residence, can be read to the subject. If it is necessary for the respondent to choose among three or more alternatives, or to give a Likert-type response, a card with the possible answers could (and most likely *should*) be given to the person so that memory will not be a factor. Open questions can be used to gather additional information, since respondents will generally give longer answers to open-ended questions verbally rather than in writing. This can sometimes be a disadvantage with verbose respondents.

Complicated questionnaires may contain items which are not appropriate for all respondents; men should not be asked how many pregnancies they have had; native-born people when they immigrated; or people who have never been hospitalized when they were last discharged. These questions are avoided with what are called 'skip patterns;' instructions or arrows indicating to the person that he or she should omit a section by skipping to a later portion of the questionnaire. Unless they are very carefully constructed and worded, skip patterns can be confusing to some respondents—and therefore likely to induce errors—if they have to follow these themselves. In contrast, interviewers, because of their training and experience in giving the questionnaire many times, can wend their way through these skip patterns much more readily, and are less likely to make mistakes. Moreover, with the advent of 'lap top' computers, the order of questions and the skip patterns can be programmed to be presented to the interviewer, so that the potential for asking the wrong questions or omitting items is minimized.

Disadvantages

Naturally, there is a cost associated with all of these advantages, in terms of both time and money. Face-to-face interviews are significantly more expensive to administer than any other method. Interviewers must be trained, so that they ask the same questions in the same way, and handle unusual circumstances similarly. In many studies, random interviews are tape-recorded, to ensure that the interviewers' styles have not changed over time; that they have not become lazy or slipshod, or sound bored. This entails further expense, for the tape-recorder itself, and for the supervisor's time to review the session and go over it with the interviewer.

If the interview is relatively short, the interviewer can arrive unannounced. This, though, takes the chance that the respondent is at home and is willing to be disturbed. The longer the session, the greater the danger that it will be seen as an imposition. For these reasons, especially when an hour or more of the person's time is needed, it is best to announce the visit beforehand, checking the respondent's willingness to participate and arranging a convenient time to come. This requirement imposes the added costs of telephoning, often repeatedly, until an answer is obtained. Further, since many people work during the day, and only evening interviews are convenient, the number of possible interviews that can be done in one day may be limited.

Another potential cost arises if, for instance, English is not the native language for a sizable proportion of the respondents. Not only must the scales and questions be translated into one or more foreign languages (as would be the case, regardless of the format), but bilingual interviewers must be found. This may not be unduly difficult if there are only a few major linguistic cultures (e.g. English and French in Quebec, Spanish in the southwestern United States, Flemish and French in Belgium), but can be more of a problem in cities which attract many immigrants from different countries. There are more languages to take into account and, if immigration has been recent, there may be few people sufficiently bilingual who can be trained as interviewers.

Finally, attributes of the interviewer may affect the responses given. This can caused by two factors: biases of the interviewer, and his or her social or ethnic characteristics (Weiss 1975). It has been known for a long time that interviewers can subtly communicate what answers they want to hear, often without being aware that they are doing so (e.g. Rice 1929). This is the easier of the two factors to deal with, since it can be overcome with adequate training (Hyman *et al.* 1954). The more difficult problem is that differences between the interviewer and respondent, especially race, also have an effect (Pettigrew 1964; Sattler 1970). Sex differences appear to play less of a role, except perhaps if sexual material is being discussed (Hyman *et al.* 1954); and age differences have not been extensively examined. Whenever possible, the race of the interviewer should be the same as that of the subject (Weiss 1975).

Telephone questionnaires

An alternative to meeting with the subjects in person is to interview them over the telephone. A major advantage is the savings incurred in terms of time and therefore money; in one Canadian study, a home interview cost $16.10, a telephone interview only $7.10 (Siemiatycki 1979). In the past, researchers have avoided this interviewing method because a significant proportion of homes did not have telephones. Moreover, this proportion was not evenly distributed, but was higher in the lower socioeconomic classes. Thus, any survey using the telephone directory as a sampling frame systematically under-represented poorer people. Indeed, the famous prediction in 1936 by the *Literary Digest* that Alf Landon would beat Roosevelt decisively was based on a telephone survey. Unfortunately for the pollsters, more Roosevelt voters than Landon voters did not have phones, leading to a biased sample.

The situation has changed considerably since then, but not always in directions that make it easier for the researcher. On the positive side, most households in North America now have telephones; in 1981, the national average in the U.S. was 93.1 per cent (Marcus and Crane 1986). However, the converse is that a larger number of people have unlisted numbers; close to 20 per cent in 1975 (Glasser and Metzger 1975). Whereas not having a telephone is still more prevalent among the lower social classes, not listing a number is, because of the additional expense, more of a middle-class phenomenon. Surprisingly, the rate of unlisted numbers among the highest income group is about the same as among the lowest (roughly 16 per cent); middle-income people have the highest unlisted rate (Glasser and Metzger 1975).

Random digit dialling

A technique has been developed to get around this problem of unlisted numbers, called *random digit dialling*. A computer-driven device dials telephone numbers at random, using either all seven digits of the number, or the last four once the three-digit exchange has been chosen by the researcher. This latter refinement was added because some exchanges consist primarily of businesses, whereas others are located in mainly residential neighbourhoods; in some areas, 80 per cent of numbers are not assigned to households (Glasser and Metzger 1972). Pre-selecting the exchange has resulted in an increase in the proportion of households reached with this technique, although it is may still not exceed 50 per cent (Waksberg 1978). One disadvantage of sampling by telephone number rather than by address or name is that homes with more than one telephone have multiple chances of being selected, a bias favouring more affluent households. Another disadvantage is that, since the selected numbers tend to be physically near one another, households tend to be more homogeneous than with a purely random sample. To overcome this 'design effect' due to cluster randomization, larger sample sizes are needed (Waksberg 1978).

Advantages

Many of the advantages of face-to-face interviewing also pertain to telephone surveys. These include (1) a reduction in the number of omitted items; (2) skip patterns are followed by the trained interviewer rather than the respondent; (3) open-ended questions can be asked; (4) a broad, representative sample can be obtained; (5) the interviewer can be prompted by a computer (a technique often referred to as CATI, or Computer Assisted Telephone Interviewing); and (6) the interviewer can determine if the person is having problems understanding the language in general or a specific question in particular.

Another advantage of telephone interviewing is that, even when the person is not willing to participate, he or she may give some basic demographic information, such as age, marital status, or education. This allows the researcher to determine if there is any systematic bias among those who decline to participate in the study.

Moreover, there are at least three areas in which the telephone may be superior to face-to-face interviews. First, any bias which may be caused by the appearance of the interviewer, due to factors such as skin colour or physical deformity, is eliminated. However, one interviewer characteristic which cannot be masked by a telephone is gender. There is some evidence that male interviewers elicit more feminist responses from women and more conservative answers from men than do female interviewers; and more optimistic reports from both sexes regarding the economic outlook (Groves and Fultz 1985). These authors also report higher refusal rates for male interviewers, which is consistent with other studies.

A second advantage is that nationwide surveys can be conducted out of one office, which lowers administrative costs and facilitates supervision of the interviewers to ensure uniformity of style. Last, there is some evidence that people may report more health-related events in a telephone interview than in a face-to-face one (Thornberry 1987), although it is not clear that the higher figure is necessarily more accurate.

Disadvantages

A potential problem with telephone interviewing is that another person in the household may be prompting the respondent. However, this risk is fairly small, since the person on the phone would have to repeat each question aloud. A more difficult issue is that there is no assurance who the person is at the other end of the line. If the sampling scheme calls for interviewing the husband, for instance, the masculine voice can be that of the chosen respondent's son or father. This may be a problem if the designated person is an immigrant unsure of his or her grasp of the language and asks a more fluent member of the household to substitute.

Another difficulty with telephone interviews, as with face-to-face ones, is that unless a specific respondent is chosen beforehand, the sample may be biased by *when* the call is made. During the day, there is a higher probability that housewives, shift workers, the ill, or the unemployed will be reached. Evening calls may similarly bias the sample by excluding shift workers. Traugott (1987) found that people reached during the day did not differ significantly from those who could be contacted only in the evening with respect to age, race, or sex; but that the latter group were more likely to be college graduates, since they tended to be employed and not work shifts.

A major problem with telephone interviewing, as opposed to face-to-face interviewing, is the difficulty with questions which require the person to choose among various options. With the interviewer present, he or she can hand the respondent a card listing the response alternatives; an option not available over the telephone. A few suggestions have been offered to overcome this problem. The easiest to implement is to have to respondent write the alternatives on a piece of paper, and then to refer to them when answering. This is feasible when one response set is used with a number of items, such as a Likert scale which will be referred to in responding to a set of questions. However, if each item requires a different list, the method can become quite tedious and demanding, and the respondent may either hang up or not write the alternatives down, relying on his or her (fallible) memory. In the latter situation, a 'primacy effect' is likely to occur, with subjects tending to endorse categories that are read toward the beginning rather than toward the end of the list (Locander and Burton 1976; Monsees and Massey 1979).

A second method is to divide the question into parts, with each section probing for a more refined answer. For example, the person can be asked if he or she agrees or disagrees with the statement. Then the next question would tap the strength of the endorsement: mild or strong. It also helps if the response format is given to the person as an introduction to the question; for example, 'In the following question, there will be four possible answers: strongly agree, mildly agree, mildly disagree, and strongly disagree. The question is . . . '.

A third method involves a pre-interview mailing to the subjects. This can consist of the entire questionnaire itself, or a card with the response alternatives. With the former, the interviewer then reads each question, with the respondent following in his or her version. The telephone call allows for probing and recording answers to open-ended questions. If a card with the alternatives is mailed, it is often combined with features like emergency telephone numbers or other items which encourage the person to keep it near the telephone, readily available when the call comes (Aneshensel *et al.* 1982).

These various techniques make it more feasible to ask complicated questions over the telephone. However, the major consideration with this form of interviewing remains to reduce complexity as much as possible. If detailed explanations are necessary, as may be the case if the person's attitudes toward public policy issues are being evaluated, face-to-face or mailed questionnaires may be preferable.

Whatever technique is used, it is highly likely that repeated calls may be necessary to reach a desired household; people may be working, out for the evening, in hospital, or on vacation. It has been recommended that three to six attempts may be required; after this, the law of diminishing returns begins to play an increasingly large role. Moreover, the call should not be made at times such that the respondents feel it would be an intrusion: on holidays, Sundays, or during major sports events.

Mailed questionnaires

Advantages

Mailing questionnaires to respondents is by far the cheapest method of the three; in Siemiatycki's study (1979), the average cost was $6.08, as opposed to $7.10 for telephone interviewing and $16.10 for home interviewing. In the past, the major drawback has been a relatively low response rate, jeopardizing the generalizability of the results. Over the years, various techniques have been developed which have resulted in higher rates of return. Dillman (1978), one of the most ardent spokesmen for this interviewing method, has combined many of them into what he calls the *Total Design Method*. He believes that response rates of over 75 per cent are possible with a general mailing to a heterogeneous population, and of 90 per cent to a targeted group, such as family practitioners.

As with telephone interviews, mailed questionnaires can be coordinated from one central office, even for national or international studies. In contrast, personal interviews usually require an office in each major city, greatly increasing the expense. Further, since there is no interviewer present, either in person or at the other end of a telephone line, social desirability bias tends to be minimized.

Disadvantages

However, there are a number of drawbacks with this method of administration. First, if a subject does not return the questionnaire, it is almost impossible to get any demographic information, obviating the possibility of comparing responders with non-responders. Second, subjects may omit some of the items; it is quite common to find statements in articles to the effect that 5 to 10 per cent of the returned questionnaires were unusable due to omitted, illegible, or invalid responses (e.g. Nelson *et al.* 1986). Third, while great care may have been taken by the investigator with regard to the sequence of the items, there is no assurance that the subjects read them in order. Some people may skip to the end first, or delay answering some questions because they have difficulty interpreting them.

A fourth difficulty is that, to ensure a high response rate (over 80 per cent), it is often necessary to send out two or three mailings to some subjects. If the identity of the respondent is known, then this necessitates some form of bookkeeping system, to record who has returned the questionnaire and who should be sent a reminder. If anonymity is desired, then reminders and additional copies must be sent to all subjects, increasing the cost of the study. Fifth, there may be a delay of up to three months until all the questionnaires that will be returned have been received. Last, there is always the possibility that some or all of the questionnaires may be delayed by a postal strike.

Increasing the return rate

Many techniques have been proposed to increase the rate of return of mailed questionnaires, although not all have proven to be effective. These have included:

1. *A covering letter.* Perhaps the most important part of a mailed questionnaire is the letter accompanying it. It will determine if the form will be looked at or thrown away, and the attitude with which the respondent will complete it. A detailed description of letters and the contents is given by Dillman (1978), who stresses their importance. The letter should begin with a statement which emphasizes two points: why the study is important; and why that person's responses are necessary to make the results interpretable, in that order. Common mistakes are to indicate in the opening paragraph that a questionnaire (a word he says is to be avoided) is enclosed; that it is part of a survey (another 'forbidden' word); identifying who the researcher is before stating why the research is being done; or under whose auspices (again, best left for later in the letter). Other points that should be included in the letter are a promise of confidentiality, a description of how the results will be used, and a mention of any incentive. The letter should

be signed by hand, with the name block under the signature indicating the person's title and affiliation. Since subjects are more likely to respond if the research is being carried out by a university or some other respected organization, its letterhead should be used whenever it is appropriate. The letter itself should fit onto one page; coloured paper may look more impressive, but does not appear to influence the response rate.

2. *Advance warning that the questionnaire will be coming.* A letter is seen as less of an intrusion than a form which has to be completed, especially one that arrives unannounced. The introductory letter thus prepares the respondent for the questionnaire, and helps differentiate it from junk mail. Unfortunately for the researcher, many 'give away' offers now use the same technique; an official-looking letter announcing the imminent arrival of a packet of chances to win millions of dollars. This makes the wording of the covering letter even more critical, in order to overcome the scepticism that often greets such unsolicited arrivals.

3. *Giving a token of appreciation in advance.* Most often, this is a nominal sum of money; the amount seems to matter less than the fact that something was given to thank the subject for his or her participation. Other incentives have included lottery tickets, pens or pencils, tie clips, unused stamps, diaries, and letter openers. If the study is done with a homogeneous group of people who may be interested in the results, a copy of the final report or paper at the conclusion of the project can be offered. The objective of these is to acknowledge that completing the questionnaire costs the person time, which is appreciated and partially compensated by the gift. It often helps to spell this out explicitly in a covering letter, indicating that the gift can be only a token of thanks.

4. *Anonymity.* The literature on the effect of anonymity on response rate is contradictory. If the person is identifiable on questionnaires which ask for confidential information, such as income, sexual practices, or illegal acts, then the response rate is definitely jeopardized. However, promises of confidentiality for non-sensitive material does not appear to materially increase compliance; although it is probably safest to ensure anonymity. If it is necessary to identify the respondent, in order to link the responses to other information or to determine who should receive follow-up reminders, then the purpose of the identification should be stated, along with guarantees that the person's name will be thrown away when it is no longer needed, and kept under lock and key in the meantime; and that in the final report, no subject will be identifiable.

5. *Personalization.* Envelopes addressed to 'Occupant' are often regarded as junk mail, and are either discarded unopened, or read in a cursory manner; the same may be true of the salutation on the letter itself. However, some people see a personalized greeting using their name as an invasion of privacy and a threat to anonymity. This problem can be handled in a

number of ways. First, the letter can be addressed to a group, such as 'Dear Colleague', 'Resident of . . . Neighbourhood', or 'Member of . . . '; the personalization is given with a handwritten signature. (Again, with the wide use by politicians and advertisers of machines which produce signatures which resemble handwriting, this may become less effective with time.) Another method to balance anonymity and personalization is to have the covering letter personalized, and to stress the fact that the questionnaire itself has no identifying information on it.

Other aspects of personalization include typed addresses rather than labels, stamps rather than metered envelopes, and regular envelopes rather than business reply ones. The former alternatives are usually associated with junk mail, and the latter with important letters. However, the individual contribution of each of these factors is still equivocal.

6. *Enclosing a stamped, self-addressed envelope.* Asking the respondents to complete the questionnaire is an imposition on their time; asking them to also find and address a return envelope and pay for the postage is a further imposition, guaranteed to lead to a high rate of non-compliance.

7. *Length of the questionnaire.* It seems logical that shorter questionnaires should lead to higher rates of return than longer ones. However, the research does not appear to bear this out. In fact, lengthening a questionnaire by adding interesting questions may actually increase compliance, indicating that once a person has been persuaded to fill out the form, its length is of secondary importance.

8. *Pre-coding the questions.* Although this does not appear to appreciably increase compliance, pre-coding does serve a number of useful purposes. First, open-ended questions must at some point be coded for analysis; in other words, coding must take place at one time or another. Second, subjects are more likely to check a box rather than write out a long explanation. Last, handwritten responses may be illegible or ambiguous. On the other hand, subjects may feel that they want to explain their answers, or indicate why none of the alternatives apply (a sign of a poorly designed question). The questionnaire can make provisions for this, having optional sections after each section or at the end for the respondent to add comments.

9. *Follow-ups.* As important as the letter introducing the study is the follow-up to maximize returns. Dillman (1978) outlines a four-step process:

- Seven to ten days after the first mailing, a postcard should be sent, thanking those who have returned the questionnaire, and reminding the others of the study's importance. The card should also indicate to those who have mislaid the original where they can get another copy of the questionnaire.
- Two to three weeks later, a second letter is sent, again emphasizing why that person's responses are necessary for this important study. Also

included are another questionnaire and return envelope. This can lead
to a problem, though, if it is sent to all subjects, irrespective of whether
or not they sent in the first form; very compliant or forgetful subjects
may complete two of them.
- The third step, which is not possible in all countries, is to send yet
  another letter, questionnaire, and envelope via registered or special
  delivery mail. The former alternative is less expensive, but some people
  may resent having to make a special trip to the post office for something
  of no direct importance to them.
- The last step, often omitted because of the expense, is to call those who
  have not responded to the previous three reminders. This may be
  impractical for studies which span the entire country, but may be feasible for more local ones.

Some researchers have maintained that while the individual effect of
each of these procedures may be slight (with the exception of the initial
letter, return envelope, and follow-up, where major effects are seen), their
cumulative effect is powerful.

The necessity of persistence

Even when all the techniques are used to maximize the return rate of a
mailed questionnaire or to talk to the designated respondent on the telephone, the initial response rate is usually too low to permit accurate conclusions to be drawn. Consequently, most surveys call for follow-up
mailings or calls in order to contact most of the subjects. The experience of
one typical telephone survey is presented in Figure 13.1, based on data
from Traugott (1987). After three follow-up calls, about two-thirds of the
respondents were contacted; one particularly elusive person required a
total of 30 calls before he was reached.

The necessity of persistence in follow-up has been demonstrated in a
number of studies which have shown that people who are easier to contact
are different in some important ways from those who are more difficult to
find or who require more reminders before they return a questionnaire.
Traugott (1987) found that during the 1984 Presidential campaign, Demo-
crats were more accessible than Republicans. As Figure 13.2 shows, people
who were found after one telephone call favoured Reagan by 3 per cent; the
lead increased to nine points when the sample included people who were
reached after three calls; and the total sample gave Reagan a 13-point advantage. He concluded that 'through persistence, the sample became younger
and more male' (p. 53). Rao (1983) and Converse and Traugott (1986) sum-
marize a number of different characteristics which are different between
early and late responders. The conclusion is that any survey is suspect

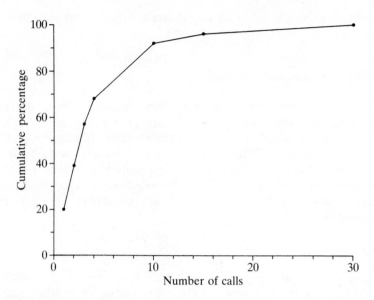

Fig. 13.1. Cumulative contact rate as a function of the number of telephone calls.

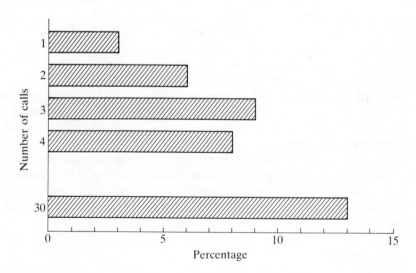

Fig. 13.2. Reagan's lead over Mondale in 1984, as a function of the number of calls required to reach the respondent.

which bases its results solely on responders to initial mailings or first telephone calls.

Computer-assisted administration

Microcomputers are now ubiquitous, found in most offices and many homes. There are now computers small enough to be placed on one's lap, which rival the power of the original mainframes. Within the past few years, it has become feasible to present even the longest questionnaires on these portable machines. Whereas just a few years ago, computer-administered questionnaires had to be given in the researcher's office, the situation has since changed, and computer-assisted interviewing (CAI) is now fairly commonplace.

Advantages

There are at least four major advantages to computerized administration. First, it can free the interviewer to do other things, or to administer the scale to a number of people simultaneously. Second, every time data are transferred from one medium to another, there is the potential for transcription and entry errors. When the subject is interviewed in person, there are many steps where these errors can creep in: the subject means to say one answer but gives another; the interviewer mishears the response; means to write one thing but puts down something else; errs in transcribing a check mark in one box to a number; or finally keys the wrong number into the computer. Having the person enter his or her responses directly into the machine eliminates all sources of error but one—unknowingly hitting the wrong key. With so many steps eliminated, there is also a commensurate saving of time and money to the researcher.

A third advantage is that neither the subject nor the interviewer can inadvertently omit items or questions. As we have already discussed, a related advantage is that the skip patterns can be automated, eliminating another source of error.

Last, people may be more honest in reporting unacceptable or undesirable behaviours to an impersonal machine than to a human. A number of studies have shown that people admit to more drinking when seated in front of a computer console than an interviewer (e.g. Lucas *et al.* 1977; Skinner and Allen 1983).

Disadvantages

One potential disadvantage of computerizing scales stems from the direct transfer of existing instruments to a computerized format. In most cases, it has not been established whether or not the translation has adversely affected their reliability and validity. Paper-and-pencil questionnaires allow subjects to see how many items there are and to pace themselves accordingly; to skip around, rather than answering the questions in sequence; and to go back easily to earlier questions, in order to change them or to check for their own consistency. While scale developers may deplore these deviations from the way the instrument was intended to be taken, the results of the original reliability and validity studies were conducted with these factors possibly playing a role. Modifying these factors *may* affect the psychometric properties of the scale; the data are not available yet (Green 1984; Moreland 1987).

A second, again potential, disadvantage is the belief, especially among health care workers, that some subjects or patients may be apprehensive about computers. These machines still retain the mystique of 'giant brains' which can, nevertheless, be brought to their knees by the press of a wrong key. However, their apprehension about subjects' reactions to these machines are probably not well founded. Most studies have found that far more people are comfortable in front of a terminal or microcomputer than are uncomfortable. Indeed, in many studies, a majority of responders preferred the machine to a human (see Stein 1987 for a review of this.) A related problem is that attitudes toward computerized interviewing may be sex-related; men tend to be more comfortable 'talking' to machines about sensitive material than to a human interviewer, while the reverse is true for women (e.g. Skinner and Allen 1983). At present, there is insufficient information to indicate whether this is due to the greater use of computers by men, or whether this attitude transcends familiarity with the machines. In either case, though, the sex difference tends to be small.

Implementation

In implementing a computerized scale or questionnaire, some considerations should be kept in mind. First, there should be an ability for the subject to interrupt the testing, and return later to the place where he or she stopped, without either losing the original data or having to go through questions already answered. This is particularly true for long scales, when it is one of many scales, or when the person may become tired or distracted easily. Second, there must be a provision for the subjects to modify their answers, both to the item they are completing at the time, and to previous ones. Respondents should be able to review their earlier answers, modify them if desired, and return to the same place in the instrument. Last, there must be a way for the subject to indicate that he or she cannot or does not want to answer a question. This option is often missing on paper-and-pencil questionnaires, since the person can simply leave the offending item out. If the subject cannot proceed to the next question without entering some response into the machine, the option must be explicit. When he was in the university town of Madison, Wisconsin, one of the pioneers in computerized interviewing, Warner Slack (cited in Fishman 1981), used the phrase 'None of your damn business' as the option the person could use to avoid a question. This was changed to 'Skip that one' when Slack moved to Boston, emphasizing the importance of cultural factors.

In summary, there is no one method of administration that is ideal in all circumstances. Factors such as cost, completion rate, and the type of question asked must all be taken into account. The final decision will, to some degree, be a compromise, in that the disadvantages of the technique that is chosen are outweighed by the positive elements.

References

Aneshensel, C. S., Frerichs, R. R., Clark, V. A., and Yokopenic, P. A. (1982). Measuring depression in the community: A comparison of telephone and personal interviews. *Public Opinion Quarterly*, **46**, 110–21.

Converse, P. E. and Traugott, M. W. (1986). Assessing the accuracy of polls and surveys. *Science*, **234**, 1094–98.

Dillman, D. A. (1978). *Mail and telephone surveys: The total design method*. Wiley, New York.

Fishman, K. D. (1981). *The computer establishment*. Harper and Row, New York.

Glasser, G. J. and Metzger, G. D. (1972). Random digit dialling as a method of telephone sampling. *Journal of Marketing Research*, **9**, 59–64.

Glasser, G. J. and Metzger, G. D. (1975). National estimates of nonlisted telephone households and their characteristics. *Journal of Marketing Research*, **12**, 359–61.

Green, B. F. (1984). *Computer-based ability testing*. American Psychological Association, Washington DC.

Groves, R. M., and Fultz, N. H. (1985). Gender effects among telephone interviewers in a survey of economic attitudes. *Sociological Methods and Research*, **14**, 31–52.

Hyman, H. H., Cobb, W. J., Feldman, J. J., Hart, C. W., and Stember, C. H. (1954). *Interviewing in social research*. University of Chicago Press, Chicago.

Locander, W. B. and Burton, J. P. (1976). The effect of question form on gathering income data by telephone. *Journal of Marketing Research*, **13**, 189–92.

Lucas, R. W., Mullin, P. J., Luna, C. B. X., and McInroy, D. C. (1977). Psychiatrists and a computer as interrogators of patients with alcohol-related illness: A comparison. *British Journal of Psychiatry*, **131**, 160–67.

Marcus, A. C. and Crane, L. A. (1986). Telephone surveys in public health research. *Medical Care*, **24**, 97–112.

Monsees, M. L. and Massey, J. T. (1979). Adapting a procedure for collecting demographic data in a personal interview to a telephone interview. *Proceedings of the American Statistical Association, Social Statistics Section*, 130–5.

Moreland, K. L. (1987). Computerized psychological assessment: What's available. In *Computerized psychological assessment* (ed. J. N. Butcher), pp. 26–49. Basic Books, New York.

Nelson, N., Rosenthal, R., and Rosnow, R. L. (1986). Interpretation of significance levels and effect sizes by psychological researchers. *American Psychologist*, **41**, 1299–301.

Pettigrew, T. F. (1964). *A profile of the Negro American*. Van Nostrand, Princeton NJ.

Quine, S. (1985). 'Does the mode matter?': A comparison of three modes of questionnaire completion. *Community Health Studies*, **9**, 151–6.

Rao, P. S. R. S. (1983). Callbacks, follow-ups, and repeated telephone calls. In *Incomplete data in sample surveys. Vol. 2: Theory and bibliographies* (eds. W. G. Madow, I. Olkin, and D. B. Rubin), pp. 33–44. Academic Press, New York.

Rice, S. A. (1929). Contagious bias in the interview. *American Journal of Sociology*, **35**, 420–3.

Sattler, J. (1970). Racial 'experimenter effects' in experimentation, interviewing and psychotherapy. *Psychological Bulletin*, **73**, 137–60.

Siemiatycki, J. (1979). A comparison of mail, telephone, and home interview strategies for household health surveys. *American Journal of Public Health*, **69**, 238–45.

Skinner, H. A. and Allen, B. A. (1983). Does the computer make a difference? Computerized versus face-to-face versus self-report assessment of alcohol, drug, and tobacco use. *Journal of Consulting and Clinical Psychology*, **51**, 267–75.

Stein, S. J. (1987) Computer-assisted diagnosis for children and adolescents. In *Computerized psychological assessment* (ed. J. N. Butcher), pp. 145–58. Basic Books, New York.

Thornberry, O. T. (1987). An experimental comparison of telephone and personal health interview surveys. *Vital and Health Statistics*. Series 2, No. 106. DHHS Pub. No. (PHS) 87-1380.

Traugott, M. W. (1987). The importance of persistence in respondent selection for preelection surveys. *Public Opinion Quarterly*, **51**, 48–57.

Waksberg, J. (1978). Sampling methods for random digit dialling. *Journal of the American Statistical Association*, **73**, 40–6.

Weiss, C. H. (1975). Interviewing in evaluation research. In *Handbook of evaluation research*, Vol. 1 (eds. E. L. Struening and M. Guttentag), pp. 355–95. Sage Publications, Beverly Hills.

Appendix A: Further reading

Chapter 1: Introduction

Colton, T. D. (1974). *Statistics in medicine*. Little Brown, Boston.
Freund, J. E. (1967). *Modern elementary statistics*. Prentice-Hall, Englewood Cliffs NJ.
Huff, D. (1954). *How to lie with statistics*. W. W. Norton, New York.
Norman, G. R. and Streiner, D. L. (1987). *PDQ statistics*. B. C. Decker, Toronto.

Chapter 2: Basic concepts

American Psychological Association (1985). *Standards for educational and psychological testing*. American Psychological Association, Washington.

Chapter 3: Developing the questions

Brislin, R. W. (1970). Back-translation for cross-cultural research. *Journal of Cross-Cultural Psychology*, **1**, 185–216.
Del Greco, L., Walop, W., and Eastridge, L. (1987). Questionnaire development: 3. Translation. *Canadian Medical Association Journal*, **136**, 817–18.
Oppenheim, A. N. (1966). *Questionnaire design and attitude measurement*. Heinemann, London.
Payne, S. L. (1951). *The art of asking questions*. Princeton University Press, Princeton NJ.
Roid, G. H. and Haladyna, T. M. (1982). *A technology for test-item writing*. Academic Press, New York.
Sudman, S. and Bradburn, N. M. (1982). *Asking questions*. Jossey-Bass, San Francisco.

Chapter 4: Scaling approaches

Dunn-Rankin, P. (1983). *Scaling methods*. Erlbaum, Hillsdale NJ.
Guilford, J. P. (1954). *Psychometric methods*. McGraw-Hill, New York.
TenBrick, T. D. (1974). *Evaluation: A practical guide for teachers*. McGraw-Hill, New York.

Chapter 5: Selecting the items

Anastasi, A. (1982). *Psychological testing* (5th edn), Chapter 8. Macmillan, New York.

Jackson, D. N. (1970). A sequential system for personality scale development. In *Current topics in clinical and community psychology* (ed. C. D. Spielberger), Vol. 2, pp. 61–96. Academic Press, New York.

Kornhauser, A. and Sheatsley, P. B. (1959). Questionnaire construction and interview procedure. In *Research methods in social relations* (eds. C. Selltiz, M. Jahoda, M. Deutsch, and S. W. Cook), rev. edn, pp. 546–87. Holt, Rinehart and Winston, New York.

Woodward, C. A., and Chambers, L. W. (1980). *Guide to questionnaire construction and question writing*. Canadian Public Health Association, Ottawa.

Chapter 6: Biases in question responses

Berg, I. A. (ed.) (1967). *Response set in personality assessment*. Aldine, Chicago.

Couch, A. and Keniston, K. (1960). Yeasayers and naysayers: Agreeing response set as a personality variable. *Journal of Abnormal and Social Psychology*, **60**, 151–74.

Edwards, A. L. (1957). *The social desirability variable in personality assessments and research*. Dryden, New York.

Thorndike, E. L. (1920). A constant error in psychological ratings. *Journal of Applied Psychology*, **4**, 25–9.

Warner, S. L. (1965). Randomized response: A survey technique for eliminating evasive answer bias. *Journal of the American Statistical Association*, **60**, 63–9.

Chapter 7: From items to scales

Nunnally, J. C., Jr. (1970). *Introduction to psychological measurement*, Chapter 8. McGraw-Hill, New York.

Chapter 8: Reliability

Anastasi, A. (1982). *Psychological testing* (5th edn), Chapter 5. Macmillan, New York.

Cronbach, L. J. (1984). *Essentials of psychological testing* (4th edn), Chapter 6. Harper and Row, New York.

Nunnally, J. C., Jr. (1970). *Introduction to psychological measurement*, Chapter 5. McGraw-Hill, New York.

Chapter 9: Generalizability theory

Brennan, R. L. (1983). *Elements of generalizability theory*. American College Testing Program, Iowa City.

Chapter 10:Validity

Anastasi, A. (1982). *Psychological testing* (5th edn). Chapters 6 and 7. Macmillan, New York.
Nunnally, J. C., Jr. (1970). *Introduction to psychological measurement*, Chapter 6. McGraw-Hill, New York.

Chapter 11: Measuring change

Nunnally, J. C., Jr. (1975). The study of change in evaluation research: Principles concerning measurement, experimental design, and analysis. In *Handbook of evaluation research* (eds. E. L. Struening and M. Guttentag), pp. 101–37. Sage, Beverly Hills.

Chapter 12: Latent-trait theories

Allen, M. J. and Yen, W. M. (1979). *Introduction to measurement theory*. Wadsworth, Belmont CA.
Bejar, I. I. (1983). *Achievement testing*. Sage, Beverly Hills.
Crocker, L. and Algina, J. (1986). *Introduction to classical and modern test theory*. Holt, Rinehart, and Winston, New York.
Hambleton, R. K. (ed.). (1983). *Applications of item response theory*. Educational Research Institute of British Columbia, Vancouver.
Lord, F. M. (1980). *Application of item response theory to practical testing problems*. Erlbaum, Hillsdale NJ.
Traub, R. E. and Wolfe, R. G. (1981). Latent trait theories and assessment of educational achievement. In *Review of research in education* 9, (ed. D. C. Berliner). American Educational Research Association, Washington DC.

Chapter 13: Methods of administration

Dillman, D. A. (1978). *Mail and telephone surveys: The total design method*. Wiley, New York.
Hyman, H. H., Cobb, W. J., Feldman, J. J., Hart, C. W., and Stember, C. H. (1954). *Interviewing in social research*. University of Chicago Press, Chicago.

Appendix B: Where to find tests

As mentioned in Chapter 3, a very useful place to find questions is to look at what others have done. Below is a partial listing of books and articles which are compendia of information about published and unpublished scales.

A. General

Backer, T. E. (1972). A reference guide for psychological measures. *Psychological Reports*, **31**, 751–68.

This article is an inventory of people, publications, and projects which may help in locating tests or information about them. It does not list any tests itself, only very useful information regarding finding them.

The mental measurements yearbooks. Buros Institute of Mental Measurements, Lincoln.

The first eight editions of the *MMY* were edited by Oscar Buros, and the set is often referred to as 'Buros'. After his death, J. V. Mitchell took over editorship of this excellent series. Only published tests are listed, and most are reviewed by two or more experts in the field. The articles also include a fairly comprehensive list of published articles and dissertations about the instruments. The yearbooks, which are not published anually, are cumulative: tests reviewed in one edition are not necessarily reviewed in subsequent ones.

The same group has also brought out more focused indices: *Reading tests and reviews*, *Tests in print*, and *Personality tests*. The latter two volumes do not have reviews, but the reader is directed back to the *MMY*.

Sweetland, R. C. and Keyser, D. J. (1986). *Tests: A comprehensive reference for assessments in psychology, education, and business* (2nd edn). Test Corporation of America, Kansas City MO.

The main volume and the *Supplement* are similar to *Tests in print*. A description is given of over 3000 published tests: purpose, format, description, appropriate population, approximate time to complete them, and where to order.

Keyser, D. J. and Sweetland, R. C. *Test critiques*. Test Corporation of America, Kansas City MO.

As of 1988, this series consists of five volumes of critical evaluations of published tests. Unlike the *MMY*, there is only one review per test, and the reference list is representative rather than exhaustive. However, the reviews tend to be considerably longer and more detailed, and follow a common format: introduction, practical applications and uses, technical aspects, and critique.

Directory of unpublished experimental mental measures. Hume Sciences Press, New York.

One of the few comprehensive sources of scales which have appeared in journals but have not been published. Volume 1 (1974) was edited by B. A. Goldman and J. L. Saunders; Volumes 2 (1978) and 3 (1982) by Goldman and J. C. Busch; and Volume 4 (1985) by Goldman and W. L. Osborne. Each test is described and one or two key articles cited. There are no reviews.

B. Social and attitudinal scales

Bonjean, C. M., Hill, R. J., and McLemore, S. D. (1967). *Sociological measurement*. Chandler, San Francisco.
Lists every scale used in four sociology journals between 1954 and 1965. Over 2000 measures are listed, with comprehensive references.

Miller, D. C. (1970). *Handbook of research design and social measurement* (2nd edn). McKay, New York.
Provides lists and examples of 36 sociometric scales in the areas of social status, group structure and dynamics, morale, job satisfaction, and the like.

Robinson, J. P., Athanasiou, R., and Head, K. B. (1969). *Measures of occupational attitudes and occupational characteristics*. Institute of Social Research, Ann Arbor.
Robinson, J. P., Rusk, J. G., and Head, K. B. (1968). *Measures of political attitude*. Institute of Social Research, Ann Arbor.
Robinson, J. P., and Shaver, P. R. (1969). *Measures of social psychological attitudes*. Institute of Social Research, Ann Arbor.
These three volumes from the ISR provide the actual items comprising the various scales. Each volume lists between 30 and 90 scales, with a short critique of each.

Shaw, M. E. and Wright, J. M. (1967). *Scales for the measurement of attitudes*. Institute of Social Research, Ann Arbor.
176 scales are described and listed, covering such areas as international and social issues, social practices and problems, political and religious attitudes, and so forth.

C. Personality

Chéné, H. (1986). *Index des variables mesurées par les tests de personalité* (2nd edn). Les Presses de l'Université Laval, Laval Quebec.
Brief, non-evaluative descriptions of primarily published tests. In French.

Chun, K-T., Cobb, S., and French, J. R. P., Jr. (1975). *Measures for psychological assessment: A guide to 3,000 original sources and their applications*. Institute of Social Research, Ann Arbor.
A listing of 3000 articles which have used various psychological tests, keyed back to the original scales.

D. Child and family

Center for the Study of Evaluation. (1970). *Elementary school test evaluations.*
Author, Los Angeles.
Center for the Study of Evaluation. (1971). *Preschool/kindergarten test evaluations.*
Author, Los Angeles.
These two volumes are designed for both professionals and school administrators.
Critical evaluations are provided for tests focused on educational objectives.

Johnson, O. G. and Bommarito, J. W. (1971). *Tests and measurements in child
development: A handbook.* Jossey-Bass, San Francisco.
This book covers over 200 tests that are not commercially published but which are
reliable and valid for children under the age of 12. A wide variety of areas are
covered, including attitudes, interests, perception, organicity, and motor skills.

Levy, P. and Goldstein, H. (eds). *Tests in education: A book of critical reviews.*
Academic Press, London.
Similar in design and intent to the *MMY* and *Test critiques*, this volume is oriented
toward published tests available in England, which do not need to be administered by a psychologist, and which cover children from nursery school through
secondary school.

Orvaschel, H., Sholomskas, D., and Weissman, M. M. (1980). *The assessment of
psychopathology and behavioral problems in children: A review of scales suitable
for epidemiological and clinical research (1967-1979).* NIMH, Rockville MD.
Orvaschel, H., and Walsh, G. (1984). *The assessment of adaptive functioning in
children: A review of existing measures suitable for epidemiological and clinical
services research.* NIMH, Rockville MD.
These two monographs list and critique unpublished scales which can be used with
children under the age of 18.

E. Health

McDowell, I. and Newell, C. (1987). *Measuring health: A guide to rating scales and
questionnaires.* Oxford University Press, Oxford.
This book reviews 50 scales in the areas of physical disability, psychological well-
being, social health, pain, and quality of life. Each scale is described in detail,
often with example questions, and its reliability and validity are reviewed. An
excellent guide.

Author index

Subject Index